FREE Study Skills Videos/DVD Offer

Dear Customer,

Thank you for your purchase from Mometrix! We consider it an honor and a privilege that you have purchased our product and we want to ensure your satisfaction.

As part of our ongoing effort to meet the needs of test takers, we have developed a set of Study Skills Videos that we would like to give you for <u>FREE</u>. These videos cover our *best practices* for getting ready for your exam, from how to use our study materials to how to best prepare for the day of the test.

All that we ask is that you email us with feedback that would describe your experience so far with our product. Good, bad, or indifferent, we want to know what you think!

To get your FREE Study Skills Videos, you can use the **QR code** below, or send us an **email** at studyvideos@mometrix.com with *FREE VIDEOS* in the subject line and the following information in the body of the email:

- The name of the product you purchased.
- Your product rating on a scale of 1-5, with 5 being the highest rating.
- Your feedback. It can be long, short, or anything in between. We just want to know your impressions and experience so far with our product. (Good feedback might include how our study material met your needs and ways we might be able to make it even better. You could highlight features that you found helpful or features that you think we should add.)

If you have any questions or concerns, please don't hesitate to contact me directly.

Thanks again!

Sincerely,

Jay Willis
Vice President
jay.willis@mometrix.com
1-800-673-8175

SCAN HERE

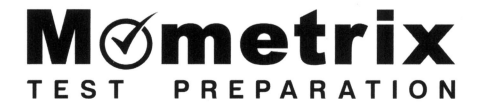

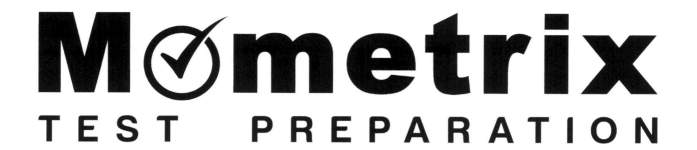

Secrets of the
Radiation
Health & Safety
Exam Study Guide

**DANB Test Review for the
Radiation Health and Safety Exam**

Written and edited by Mometrix Test Prep

Printed in the United States of America

This paper meets the requirements of ANSI/NISO Z39.48-1992 (Permanence of Paper).

Mometrix offers volume discount pricing to institutions. For more information or a price quote, please contact our sales department at sales@mometrix.com or 888-248-1219.

Paperback
ISBN 13: 978-1-60971-616-5
ISBN 10: 1-6097-1616-7

DEAR FUTURE EXAM SUCCESS STORY

First of all, **THANK YOU** for purchasing Mometrix study materials!

Second, congratulations! You are one of the few determined test-takers who are committed to doing whatever it takes to excel on your exam. **You have come to the right place.** We developed these study materials with one goal in mind: to deliver you the information you need in a format that's concise and easy to use.

In addition to optimizing your guide for the content of the test, we've outlined our recommended steps for breaking down the preparation process into small, attainable goals so you can make sure you stay on track.

We've also analyzed the entire test-taking process, identifying the most common pitfalls and showing how you can overcome them and be ready for any curveball the test throws you.

Standardized testing is one of the biggest obstacles on your road to success, which only increases the importance of doing well in the high-pressure, high-stakes environment of test day. Your results on this test could have a significant impact on your future, and this guide provides the information and practical advice to help you achieve your full potential on test day.

Your success is our success

We would love to hear from you! If you would like to share the story of your exam success or if you have any questions or comments in regard to our products, please contact us at **800-673-8175** or **support@mometrix.com**.

Thanks again for your business and we wish you continued success!

Sincerely,
The Mometrix Test Preparation Team

Need more help? Check out our flashcards at:
http://mometrixflashcards.com/DANB

TABLE OF CONTENTS

Introduction

Thank you for purchasing this resource! You have made the choice to prepare yourself for a test that could have a huge impact on your future, and this guide is designed to help you be fully ready for test day. Obviously, it's important to have a solid understanding of the test material, but you also need to be prepared for the unique environment and stressors of the test, so that you can perform to the best of your abilities.

For this purpose, the first section that appears in this guide is the **Secret Keys**. We've devoted countless hours to meticulously researching what works and what doesn't, and we've boiled down our findings to the five most impactful steps you can take to improve your performance on the test. We start at the beginning with study planning and move through the preparation process, all the way to the testing strategies that will help you get the most out of what you know when you're finally sitting in front of the test.

We recommend that you start preparing for your test as far in advance as possible. However, if you've bought this guide as a last-minute study resource and only have a few days before your test, we recommend that you skip over the first two Secret Keys since they address a long-term study plan.

If you struggle with **test anxiety**, we strongly encourage you to check out our recommendations for how you can overcome it. Test anxiety is a formidable foe, but it can be beaten, and we want to make sure you have the tools you need to defeat it.

Secret Key #1 – Plan Big, Study Small

There's a lot riding on your performance. If you want to ace this test, you're going to need to keep your skills sharp and the material fresh in your mind. You need a plan that lets you review everything you need to know while still fitting in your schedule. We'll break this strategy down into three categories.

Information Organization

Start with the information you already have: the official test outline. From this, you can make a complete list of all the concepts you need to cover before the test. Organize these concepts into groups that can be studied together, and create a list of any related vocabulary you need to learn so you can brush up on any difficult terms. You'll want to keep this vocabulary list handy once you actually start studying since you may need to add to it along the way.

Time Management

Once you have your set of study concepts, decide how to spread them out over the time you have left before the test. Break your study plan into small, clear goals so you have a manageable task for each day and know exactly what you're doing. Then just focus on one small step at a time. When you manage your time this way, you don't need to spend hours at a time studying. Studying a small block of content for a short period each day helps you retain information better and avoid stressing over how much you have left to do. You can relax knowing that you have a plan to cover everything in time. In order for this strategy to be effective though, you have to start studying early and stick to your schedule. Avoid the exhaustion and futility that comes from last-minute cramming!

Study Environment

The environment you study in has a big impact on your learning. Studying in a coffee shop, while probably more enjoyable, is not likely to be as fruitful as studying in a quiet room. It's important to keep distractions to a minimum. You're only planning to study for a short block of time, so make the most of it. Don't pause to check your phone or get up to find a snack. It's also important to **avoid multitasking**. Research has consistently shown that multitasking will make your studying dramatically less effective. Your study area should also be comfortable and well-lit so you don't have the distraction of straining your eyes or sitting on an uncomfortable chair.

 The time of day you study is also important. You want to be rested and alert. Don't wait until just before bedtime. Study when you'll be most likely to comprehend and remember. Even better, if you know what time of day your test will be, set that time aside for study. That way your brain will be used to working on that subject at that specific time and you'll have a better chance of recalling information.

Finally, it can be helpful to team up with others who are studying for the same test. Your actual studying should be done in as isolated an environment as possible, but the work of organizing the information and setting up the study plan can be divided up. In between study sessions, you can discuss with your teammates the concepts that you're all studying and quiz each other on the details. Just be sure that your teammates are as serious about the test as you are. If you find that your study time is being replaced with social time, you might need to find a new team.

Secret Key #2 – Make Your Studying Count

You're devoting a lot of time and effort to preparing for this test, so you want to be absolutely certain it will pay off. This means doing more than just reading the content and hoping you can remember it on test day. It's important to make every minute of study count. There are two main areas you can focus on to make your studying count.

Retention

It doesn't matter how much time you study if you can't remember the material. You need to make sure you are retaining the concepts. To check your retention of the information you're learning, try recalling it at later times with minimal prompting. Try carrying around flashcards and glance at one or two from time to time or ask a friend who's also studying for the test to quiz you.

To enhance your retention, look for ways to put the information into practice so that you can apply it rather than simply recalling it. If you're using the information in practical ways, it will be much easier to remember. Similarly, it helps to solidify a concept in your mind if you're not only reading it to yourself but also explaining it to someone else. Ask a friend to let you teach them about a concept you're a little shaky on (or speak aloud to an imaginary audience if necessary). As you try to summarize, define, give examples, and answer your friend's questions, you'll understand the concepts better and they will stay with you longer. Finally, step back for a big picture view and ask yourself how each piece of information fits with the whole subject. When you link the different concepts together and see them working together as a whole, it's easier to remember the individual components.

Finally, practice showing your work on any multi-step problems, even if you're just studying. Writing out each step you take to solve a problem will help solidify the process in your mind, and you'll be more likely to remember it during the test.

Modality

Modality simply refers to the means or method by which you study. Choosing a study modality that fits your own individual learning style is crucial. No two people learn best in exactly the same way, so it's important to know your strengths and use them to your advantage.

For example, if you learn best by visualization, focus on visualizing a concept in your mind and draw an image or a diagram. Try color-coding your notes, illustrating them, or creating symbols that will trigger your mind to recall a learned concept. If you learn best by hearing or discussing information, find a study partner who learns the same way or read aloud to yourself. Think about how to put the information in your own words. Imagine that you are giving a lecture on the topic and record yourself so you can listen to it later.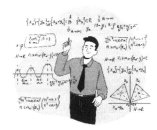

For any learning style, flashcards can be helpful. Organize the information so you can take advantage of spare moments to review. Underline key words or phrases. Use different colors for different categories. Mnemonic devices (such as creating a short list in which every item starts with the same letter) can also help with retention. Find what works best for you and use it to store the information in your mind most effectively and easily.

3

Secret Key #3 – Practice the Right Way

Your success on test day depends not only on how many hours you put into preparing, but also on whether you prepared the right way. It's good to check along the way to see if your studying is paying off. One of the most effective ways to do this is by taking practice tests to evaluate your progress. Practice tests are useful because they show exactly where you need to improve. Every time you take a practice test, pay special attention to these three groups of questions:

- The questions you got wrong
- The questions you had to guess on, even if you guessed right
- The questions you found difficult or slow to work through

This will show you exactly what your weak areas are, and where you need to devote more study time. Ask yourself why each of these questions gave you trouble. Was it because you didn't understand the material? Was it because you didn't remember the vocabulary? Do you need more repetitions on this type of question to build speed and confidence? Dig into those questions and figure out how you can strengthen your weak areas as you go back to review the material.

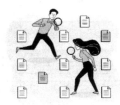 Additionally, many practice tests have a section explaining the answer choices. It can be tempting to read the explanation and think that you now have a good understanding of the concept. However, an explanation likely only covers part of the question's broader context. Even if the explanation makes perfect sense, **go back and investigate** every concept related to the question until you're positive you have a thorough understanding.

As you go along, keep in mind that the practice test is just that: practice. Memorizing these questions and answers will not be very helpful on the actual test because it is unlikely to have any of the same exact questions. If you only know the right answers to the sample questions, you won't be prepared for the real thing. **Study the concepts** until you understand them fully, and then you'll be able to answer any question that shows up on the test.

It's important to wait on the practice tests until you're ready. If you take a test on your first day of study, you may be overwhelmed by the amount of material covered and how much you need to learn. Work up to it gradually.

On test day, you'll need to be prepared for answering questions, managing your time, and using the test-taking strategies you've learned. It's a lot to balance, like a mental marathon that will have a big impact on your future. Like training for a marathon, you'll need to start slowly and work your way up. When test day arrives, you'll be ready.

Start with the strategies you've read in the first two Secret Keys—plan your course and study in the way that works best for you. If you have time, consider using multiple study resources to get different approaches to the same concepts. It can be helpful to see difficult concepts from more than one angle. Then find a good source for practice tests. Many times, the test website will suggest potential study resources or provide sample tests.

Practice Test Strategy

If you're able to find at least three practice tests, we recommend this strategy:

UNTIMED AND OPEN-BOOK PRACTICE

Take the first test with no time constraints and with your notes and study guide handy. Take your time and focus on applying the strategies you've learned.

TIMED AND OPEN-BOOK PRACTICE

Take the second practice test open-book as well, but set a timer and practice pacing yourself to finish in time.

TIMED AND CLOSED-BOOK PRACTICE

Take any other practice tests as if it were test day. Set a timer and put away your study materials. Sit at a table or desk in a quiet room, imagine yourself at the testing center, and answer questions as quickly and accurately as possible.

Keep repeating timed and closed-book tests on a regular basis until you run out of practice tests or it's time for the actual test. Your mind will be ready for the schedule and stress of test day, and you'll be able to focus on recalling the material you've learned.

Secret Key #4 – Pace Yourself

Once you're fully prepared for the material on the test, your biggest challenge on test day will be managing your time. Just knowing that the clock is ticking can make you panic even if you have plenty of time left. Work on pacing yourself so you can build confidence against the time constraints of the exam. Pacing is a difficult skill to master, especially in a high-pressure environment, so **practice is vital**.

Set time expectations for your pace based on how much time is available. For example, if a section has 60 questions and the time limit is 30 minutes, you know you have to average 30 seconds or less per question in order to answer them all. Although 30 seconds is the hard limit, set 25 seconds per question as your goal, so you reserve extra time to spend on harder questions. When you budget extra time for the harder questions, you no longer have any reason to stress when those questions take longer to answer.

Don't let this time expectation distract you from working through the test at a calm, steady pace, but keep it in mind so you don't spend too much time on any one question. Recognize that taking extra time on one question you don't understand may keep you from answering two that you do understand later in the test. If your time limit for a question is up and you're still not sure of the answer, mark it and move on, and come back to it later if the time and the test format allow. If the testing format doesn't allow you to return to earlier questions, just make an educated guess; then put it out of your mind and move on.

On the easier questions, be careful not to rush. It may seem wise to hurry through them so you have more time for the challenging ones, but it's not worth missing one if you know the concept and just didn't take the time to read the question fully. Work efficiently but make sure you understand the question and have looked at all of the answer choices, since more than one may seem right at first.

Even if you're paying attention to the time, you may find yourself a little behind at some point. You should speed up to get back on track, but do so wisely. Don't panic; just take a few seconds less on each question until you're caught up. Don't guess without thinking, but do look through the answer choices and eliminate any you know are wrong. If you can get down to two choices, it is often worthwhile to guess from those. Once you've chosen an answer, move on and don't dwell on any that you skipped or had to hurry through. If a question was taking too long, chances are it was one of the harder ones, so you weren't as likely to get it right anyway.

On the other hand, if you find yourself getting ahead of schedule, it may be beneficial to slow down a little. The more quickly you work, the more likely you are to make a careless mistake that will affect your score. You've budgeted time for each question, so don't be afraid to spend that time. Practice an efficient but careful pace to get the most out of the time you have.

Secret Key #5 – Have a Plan for Guessing

When you're taking the test, you may find yourself stuck on a question. Some of the answer choices seem better than others, but you don't see the one answer choice that is obviously correct. What do you do?

The scenario described above is very common, yet most test takers have not effectively prepared for it. Developing and practicing a plan for guessing may be one of the single most effective uses of your time as you get ready for the exam.

In developing your plan for guessing, there are three questions to address:

- When should you start the guessing process?
- How should you narrow down the choices?
- Which answer should you choose?

When to Start the Guessing Process

Unless your plan for guessing is to select C every time (which, despite its merits, is not what we recommend), you need to leave yourself enough time to apply your answer elimination strategies. Since you have a limited amount of time for each question, that means that if you're going to give yourself the best shot at guessing correctly, you have to decide quickly whether or not you will guess.

Of course, the best-case scenario is that you don't have to guess at all, so first, see if you can answer the question based on your knowledge of the subject and basic reasoning skills. Focus on the key words in the question and try to jog your memory of related topics. Give yourself a chance to bring the knowledge to mind, but once you realize that you don't have (or you can't access) the knowledge you need to answer the question, it's time to start the guessing process.

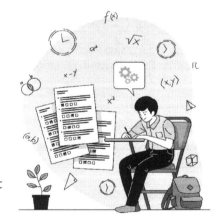

It's almost always better to start the guessing process too early than too late. It only takes a few seconds to remember something and answer the question from knowledge. Carefully eliminating wrong answer choices takes longer. Plus, going through the process of eliminating answer choices can actually help jog your memory.

Summary: Start the guessing process as soon as you decide that you can't answer the question based on your knowledge.

7

How to Narrow Down the Choices

The next chapter in this book (**Test-Taking Strategies**) includes a wide range of strategies for how to approach questions and how to look for answer choices to eliminate. You will definitely want to read those carefully, practice them, and figure out which ones work best for you. Here though, we're going to address a mindset rather than a particular strategy.

Your odds of guessing an answer correctly depend on how many options you are choosing from.

Number of options left	5	4	3	2	1
Odds of guessing correctly	20%	25%	33%	50%	100%

You can see from this chart just how valuable it is to be able to eliminate incorrect answers and make an educated guess, but there are two things that many test takers do that cause them to miss out on the benefits of guessing:

- Accidentally eliminating the correct answer
- Selecting an answer based on an impression

We'll look at the first one here, and the second one in the next section.

To avoid accidentally eliminating the correct answer, we recommend a thought exercise called **the $5 challenge**. In this challenge, you only eliminate an answer choice from contention if you are willing to bet $5 on it being wrong. Why $5? Five dollars is a small but not insignificant amount of money. It's an amount you could afford to lose but wouldn't want to throw away. And while losing

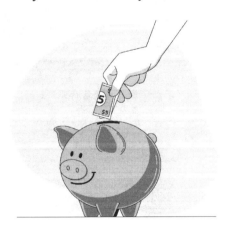

$5 once might not hurt too much, doing it twenty times will set you back $100. In the same way, each small decision you make—eliminating a choice here, guessing on a question there—won't by itself impact your score very much, but when you put them all together, they can make a big difference. By holding each answer choice elimination decision to a higher standard, you can reduce the risk of accidentally eliminating the correct answer.

The $5 challenge can also be applied in a positive sense: If you are willing to bet $5 that an answer choice *is* correct, go ahead and mark it as correct.

Summary: Only eliminate an answer choice if you are willing to bet $5 that it is wrong.

Which Answer to Choose

You're taking the test. You've run into a hard question and decided you'll have to guess. You've eliminated all the answer choices you're willing to bet $5 on. Now you have to pick an answer. Why do we even need to talk about this? Why can't you just pick whichever one you feel like when the time comes?

The answer to these questions is that if you don't come into the test with a plan, you'll rely on your impression to select an answer choice, and if you do that, you risk falling into a trap. The test writers know that everyone who takes their test will be guessing on some of the questions, so they intentionally write wrong answer choices to seem plausible. You still have to pick an answer though, and if the wrong answer choices are designed to look right, how can you ever be sure that you're not falling for their trap? The best solution we've found to this dilemma is to take the decision out of your hands entirely. Here is the process we recommend:

Once you've eliminated any choices that you are confident (willing to bet $5) are wrong, select the first remaining choice as your answer.

Whether you choose to select the first remaining choice, the second, or the last, the important thing is that you use some preselected standard. Using this approach guarantees that you will not be enticed into selecting an answer choice that looks right, because you are not basing your decision on how the answer choices look.

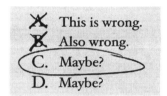

This is not meant to make you question your knowledge. Instead, it is to help you recognize the difference between your knowledge and your impressions. There's a huge difference between thinking an answer is right because of what you know, and thinking an answer is right because it looks or sounds like it should be right.

Summary: To ensure that your selection is appropriately random, make a predetermined selection from among all answer choices you have not eliminated.

Test-Taking Strategies

This section contains a list of test-taking strategies that you may find helpful as you work through the test. By taking what you know and applying logical thought, you can maximize your chances of answering any question correctly!

It is very important to realize that every question is different and every person is different: no single strategy will work on every question, and no single strategy will work for every person. That's why we've included all of them here, so you can try them out and determine which ones work best for different types of questions and which ones work best for you.

Question Strategies

✓ READ CAREFULLY

Read the question and the answer choices carefully. Don't miss the question because you misread the terms. You have plenty of time to read each question thoroughly and make sure you understand what is being asked. Yet a happy medium must be attained, so don't waste too much time. You must read carefully and efficiently.

✓ CONTEXTUAL CLUES

Look for contextual clues. If the question includes a word you are not familiar with, look at the immediate context for some indication of what the word might mean. Contextual clues can often give you all the information you need to decipher the meaning of an unfamiliar word. Even if you can't determine the meaning, you may be able to narrow down the possibilities enough to make a solid guess at the answer to the question.

✓ PREFIXES

If you're having trouble with a word in the question or answer choices, try dissecting it. Take advantage of every clue that the word might include. Prefixes can be a huge help. Usually, they allow you to determine a basic meaning. *Pre-* means before, *post-* means after, *pro-* is positive, *de-* is negative. From prefixes, you can get an idea of the general meaning of the word and try to put it into context.

✓ HEDGE WORDS

Watch out for critical hedge words, such as *likely, may, can, sometimes, often, almost, mostly, usually, generally, rarely*, and *sometimes*. Question writers insert these hedge phrases to cover every possibility. Often an answer choice will be wrong simply because it leaves no room for exception. Be on guard for answer choices that have definitive words such as *exactly* and *always*.

✓ SWITCHBACK WORDS

Stay alert for *switchbacks*. These are the words and phrases frequently used to alert you to shifts in thought. The most common switchback words are *but, although*, and *however*. Others include *nevertheless, on the other hand, even though, while, in spite of, despite*, and *regardless of*. Switchback words are important to catch because they can change the direction of the question or an answer choice.

10

⌀ FACE VALUE

When in doubt, use common sense. Accept the situation in the problem at face value. Don't read too much into it. These problems will not require you to make wild assumptions. If you have to go beyond creativity and warp time or space in order to have an answer choice fit the question, then you should move on and consider the other answer choices. These are normal problems rooted in reality. The applicable relationship or explanation may not be readily apparent, but it is there for you to figure out. Use your common sense to interpret anything that isn't clear.

Answer Choice Strategies

⌀ ANSWER SELECTION

The most thorough way to pick an answer choice is to identify and eliminate wrong answers until only one is left, then confirm it is the correct answer. Sometimes an answer choice may immediately seem right, but be careful. The test writers will usually put more than one reasonable answer choice on each question, so take a second to read all of them and make sure that the other choices are not equally obvious. As long as you have time left, it is better to read every answer choice than to pick the first one that looks right without checking the others.

⌀ ANSWER CHOICE FAMILIES

An answer choice family consists of two (in rare cases, three) answer choices that are very similar in construction and cannot all be true at the same time. If you see two answer choices that are direct opposites or parallels, one of them is usually the correct answer. For instance, if one answer choice says that quantity x increases and another either says that quantity x decreases (opposite) or says that quantity y increases (parallel), then those answer choices would fall into the same family. An answer choice that doesn't match the construction of the answer choice family is more likely to be incorrect. Most questions will not have answer choice families, but when they do appear, you should be prepared to recognize them.

⌀ ELIMINATE ANSWERS

Eliminate answer choices as soon as you realize they are wrong, but make sure you consider all possibilities. If you are eliminating answer choices and realize that the last one you are left with is also wrong, don't panic. Start over and consider each choice again. There may be something you missed the first time that you will realize on the second pass.

⌀ AVOID FACT TRAPS

Don't be distracted by an answer choice that is factually true but doesn't answer the question. You are looking for the choice that answers the question. Stay focused on what the question is asking for so you don't accidentally pick an answer that is true but incorrect. Always go back to the question and make sure the answer choice you've selected actually answers the question and is not merely a true statement.

⌀ EXTREME STATEMENTS

In general, you should avoid answers that put forth extreme actions as standard practice or proclaim controversial ideas as established fact. An answer choice that states the "process should be used in certain situations, if..." is much more likely to be correct than one that states the "process should be discontinued completely." The first is a calm rational statement and doesn't even make a definitive, uncompromising stance, using a hedge word *if* to provide wiggle room, whereas the second choice is far more extreme.

☑ Benchmark

As you read through the answer choices and you come across one that seems to answer the question well, mentally select that answer choice. This is not your final answer, but it's the one that will help you evaluate the other answer choices. The one that you selected is your benchmark or standard for judging each of the other answer choices. Every other answer choice must be compared to your benchmark. That choice is correct until proven otherwise by another answer choice beating it. If you find a better answer, then that one becomes your new benchmark. Once you've decided that no other choice answers the question as well as your benchmark, you have your final answer.

☑ Predict the Answer

Before you even start looking at the answer choices, it is often best to try to predict the answer. When you come up with the answer on your own, it is easier to avoid distractions and traps because you will know exactly what to look for. The right answer choice is unlikely to be word-for-word what you came up with, but it should be a close match. Even if you are confident that you have the right answer, you should still take the time to read each option before moving on.

General Strategies

☑ Tough Questions

If you are stumped on a problem or it appears too hard or too difficult, don't waste time. Move on! Remember though, if you can quickly check for obviously incorrect answer choices, your chances of guessing correctly are greatly improved. Before you completely give up, at least try to knock out a couple of possible answers. Eliminate what you can and then guess at the remaining answer choices before moving on.

☑ Check Your Work

Since you will probably not know every term listed and the answer to every question, it is important that you get credit for the ones that you do know. Don't miss any questions through careless mistakes. If at all possible, try to take a second to look back over your answer selection and make sure you've selected the correct answer choice and haven't made a costly careless mistake (such as marking an answer choice that you didn't mean to mark). This quick double check should more than pay for itself in caught mistakes for the time it costs.

☑ Pace Yourself

It's easy to be overwhelmed when you're looking at a page full of questions; your mind is confused and full of random thoughts, and the clock is ticking down faster than you would like. Calm down and maintain the pace that you have set for yourself. Especially as you get down to the last few minutes of the test, don't let the small numbers on the clock make you panic. As long as you are on track by monitoring your pace, you are guaranteed to have time for each question.

☑ Don't Rush

It is very easy to make errors when you are in a hurry. Maintaining a fast pace in answering questions is pointless if it makes you miss questions that you would have gotten right otherwise. Test writers like to include distracting information and wrong answers that seem right. Taking a little extra time to avoid careless mistakes can make all the difference in your test score. Find a pace that allows you to be confident in the answers that you select.

12

⊘ Keep Moving

Panicking will not help you pass the test, so do your best to stay calm and keep moving. Taking deep breaths and going through the answer elimination steps you practiced can help to break through a stress barrier and keep your pace.

Final Notes

The combination of a solid foundation of content knowledge and the confidence that comes from practicing your plan for applying that knowledge is the key to maximizing your performance on test day. As your foundation of content knowledge is built up and strengthened, you'll find that the strategies included in this chapter become more and more effective in helping you quickly sift through the distractions and traps of the test to isolate the correct answer.

Now that you're preparing to move forward into the test content chapters of this book, be sure to keep your goal in mind. As you read, think about how you will be able to apply this information on the test. If you've already seen sample questions for the test and you have an idea of the question format and style, try to come up with questions of your own that you can answer based on what you're reading. This will give you valuable practice applying your knowledge in the same ways you can expect to on test day.

Good luck and good studying!

Purpose and Technique

Transform passive reading into active learning! After immersing yourself in this chapter, put your comprehension to the test by taking a quiz. The insights you gained will stay with you longer this way. Scan the QR code to go directly to the chapter quiz interface for this study guide. If you're using a computer, simply visit the bonus page at **mometrix.com/bonus948/danbrhs** and click the Chapter Quizzes link.

Anatomical Landmarks, Conditions, and Materials

ORAL CAVITY VARIATIONS

A number of anatomical variations or **sensitivities** that may be present in the oral cavity can affect the use of radiography. The positioning of the sensor is difficult for shots of the lower jaw in individuals with large tongues, for example. If the roof of the mouth is shallow, it may be difficult to maintain a parallel relationship between the sensor and the long axes of the teeth in the upper jaw. This is because the digital sensors are rigid and do not allow for any bending or flexing. For that reason, the sensor must be placed in a manner where it fits into the oral cavity combined with proper use of the bisecting or paralleling technique. Vertical angulation may need to be increased, which increases the probability of a foreshortened image. There are several types of common bony outgrowths or exostoses that can create problems. About one-fifth of the population has this type of growth in the middle of their hard palate (torus palatinus) and a smaller proportion of people have similar growths on the lower jaw (torus mandibularis). In both cases, the rigid sensor should not be placed over the bony growth as this can be painful for the patient and cause distortion on the resulting image. Some people have very sensitive mucous membranes or high muscle attachments in the area around the premolars of the lower jaw, and the sensor placement may need to be adjusted accordingly to prevent impingement on the tissue. Sensitivity in the mandibular incisor area is also common when exposing dental images due to the corners of the sensor pinching the soft mucous membranes of the floor of the mouth. Lastly, some patients will be fully or partially edentulous, and exposure times for these individuals can be minimal.

IMPLANT THERAPY

When sites for possible dental implants are selected, it is necessary to know the amount of bone present and the position of certain anatomical structures. Numerous images of the area are needed. Tomography should be used to assess and obtain a three-dimensional view of various sites. Two different cuts, cross-sectional and sagittal, may be traced with linear tomography. Alternatively, computed tomography or a CT scan can be utilized. CT has some disadvantages including high cost, augmented radiation exposure, obscuration by artifacts, or general lack of image detail. In reality, many dental practices do not use tomography for assessment of implant therapy, substituting a combination of other types of radiographs. These substitutions are not recommended because they do not give accurate three-dimensional views.

IMPROVING EXPOSURE OF THIRD MOLARS

It can be challenging to obtain diagnostic images of third molars, and often extraoral or panoramic views must be taken. The major problem with normal intraoral exposures of the upper jaw is excitation of the gag reflex. A RINN or Snap-A-Ray are commonly used to keep the sensor away from the palate. This combined with an increased vertical angulation minimizes spatial errors. In

15

the mandible, it can be challenging to place the sensor far enough back in the mouth, so techniques to relax the muscle on the floor of the mouth, move the tongue to the side, and/or direct the beam from the distal side are usually employed.

ENDODONTIC PROBLEMS

Individuals undergoing management of endodontic or pulp problems will be treated with the use of a dental dam isolating the affected tooth/teeth in the oral cavity. The best way to take a radiograph is to remove the frame of the dam and position the sensor with a RINN XCP positioning device. The patient can assist by holding the RINN XCP device in a manner that positions the sensor parallel to the tooth. The exposure should be captured very quickly.

TRISMUS

Patients with infections or some type of injury may be unable to open their mouth to some extent due to a condition called trismus. Diagnostic radiographs are usually indicated in these individuals. If possible, intraoral exposures can be taken by inserting and orienting the sensor with a RINN XCP device. There are a number of different types of RINN XCP devices available to allow for various levels of trismus. If it is determined that a patient is unable to tolerate the intraoral sensor or RINN XCP device, the dental team may utilize an extraoral technique to obtain a view of the affected area.

EDENTULOUS PATIENTS

Edentulous patients have partial or complete areas in their mouth where there are no teeth. They may also have pathological abnormalities like infected areas, cysts, remnants of roots, or unerupted or extra teeth. If possible, a panoramic survey should be performed on edentulous patients as this type of imaging can capture large portions of the oral cavity and surrounding areas. If a panoramic image is not possible, a series of 10 to14 periapical images using a size 2 digital sensor can be taken, which will allow the dentist to view the alveolar bone throughout the oral cavity. Similar to dentulous patients, the paralleling technique can be used on edentulous patients without significant bone resorption. When the bone levels are minimal and unable to properly angle the RINN XCP and the digital sensor bisecting imaging method can be used.

THE TEMPOROMANDIBULAR JOINT

The TMJ or temporomandibular joints connects the mandible to the temporal bones on both sides of the skull. Visualization of the TMJ region is diagnostic for a number of problems including popping and clicking of the jaw as well as conditions such as trismus and clenching of the teeth. The radiographic techniques utilized to capture the TMJ area are very specialized and generally are performed outside the normal dental practice. In a normal dental office, the only types of TMJ analysis usually available are either transcranial lateral projections or specialized adaptations of panoramic projections. A transcranial lateral view obliquely angles the center of the x-ray beam from above toward the condyle on the opposing side; the image is usually quite distorted and does not pick up some vital diagnostic areas. Specialized panoramic projections can be used to pick up obvious changes, but the beam can only be directed obliquely to the axis of the condyle which limits the utility of this technique as well. Sometimes submentovertex projections, where the beam is directed from below the chin, are used to observe TMJ.

TMJ TOMOGRAPHY

The TMJ region is usually documented in specialized facilities that have machines to perform analysis beyond the standard periapical and panoramic projections. One of the techniques used to capture the TMJ area is TMJ tomography. The principle involved is similar to panoramic radiography in that an x-ray tube and sensor are rotating in opposite directions around a central fixed point in this case. The focal plane is primarily visualized, and the rest is blurry. The thickness

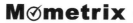

of the focal plane is controlled by the angle between shots, and its position is influenced by the position of the central fulcrum. The relationship between the tube and sensor can be linear or in some other trajectory like circular, elliptical, or cloverleaf. CT scanning is a type of tomography that uses digital imagery; the method is more expensive but can provide finer details.

Use of MRI

Magnetic resonance imaging or MRI can be employed to visualize the TMJ or other areas without the use of ionizing radiation. It is the only technique that can document all areas related to TMJ functional abnormalities, including the discs and rear attachments of the temporomandibular joints, the condyle, and the fossae or groove of the lower jaw. In MRI, the individual is subjected to a magnetic field. Atoms of hydrogen in the body are realigned by the electromagnetic forces generated. After the area being documented is subsequently bombarded with radio frequency waves, the protons release the energy absorbed. A sensor picks up this information and sends it to a computer which provides an image. The technique is especially useful for visualization of soft tissues.

Developmental Abnormalities That Affect Sensor Placement

If an individual has a **narrow dental arch**, it may be necessary to use a smaller sensor size, typically size 0 or 1 to capture images in the front of the mouth. If the patient has a **shallow palatial vault**, it may be difficult to place the RINN XCP with the sensor in the correct position using the paralleling method; solutions include use of a size 1 sensor size or the bisecting technique. Some people have **stiff lingual tongue attachments**, which make it difficult to place the sensor near the floor of the mouth; here the bisecting-angle technique is generally used. If a patient has a **bony ridge or torus in the mandible**, the sensor and the RINN XCP must be placed on the far side of the tori, adjusting the vertical angulation to balance the larger angle between the sensor and the long axis of the tooth. Presence of an **oversized palatial cusp** at the first premolar of the maxilla is a widespread abnormality. In these cases, the canine will appear to be overlapped unless the direction of the x-ray beam is more distal.

Radiographic Surveys for Pediatric Patients

The importance of capturing dental images on pediatric patients is essential not only to evaluate the health of the teeth in the primary dentition, but also to provide an early diagnosis and develop an early treatment plan for any anomalies or pathological conditions. Similar to adults, pediatric patients can experience dental cysts, tumors and other malignancies that can only be detected with dental images including the panoramic technique and both the periapical and bitewing technique. Children with genetic predisposition or other risk factors for caries should have posterior bitewings taken as the primary teeth erupt and enter the functional dentition phase Bitewings are generally done every year to 1 ½ years until permanent teeth come when the interval can be lengthened to 2 years. The interval can also be shortened in the event a pediatric patient exhibits chronic decay patterns as a method of evaluating the treatment plan and patients home care.

Guidelines

When considering the type of dental image to capture on a pediatric patient, the panoramic technique is the preferred technique as it exposes the patient to less radiation and can capture a larger area of the mouth. New technology often allows the panoramic machine to create supplemental bitewing images from the original panoramic image without any additional radiation exposure to the patient. If a panoramic machine is unavailable, the types of radiographs taken should depend on the child's age or dentition. Surveys for young children in the early eruptive stage (usually up to 5 years of age) generally consist of occlusal image of both the maxillary and mandibular arch as well as periapical and bitewing projections. Because pediatric patients typically

17

have smaller mouths, the dental team may choose a size 0 or 1 digital sensor to capture periapical and/or bitewing images. Between about 6 and 9 years of age, pediatric patients tend to be in the mixed dentition phase with both primary and permanent teeth found in the mouth. In this age range, the radiographic documentation generally resembles a regular full-mouth survey with the exception that a size 1 sensor may be used for periapical images and a size 2 sensor for posterior bitewings. Pediatric patients in the older preadolescent group, about 10-12 years old, commonly have a full mouth series captured which includes 14 periapical images and 4 bitewing images.

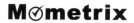

Purposes of Radiographic Images

INTRAORAL RADIOGRAPHS

There are three types of intraoral radiographs:

- **Periapical radiographs** are used to display the location, outlines, and distance from the central jaw arch of the teeth into the surrounding tissue area. The entire tooth and root of all required teeth on a given periapical, including minimally 2 mm of the periapical bone below the apex of the teeth, are required. Sensor positioning devices such as the RINN XCP or Snap-a-Ray are utilized during periapical exposures.
- **Bitewing radiographs** are used to show the entire coronal portion of the tooth or at a minimum, the visible part of the tooth covered by enamel as well as a surrounding bone. Bitewing images are useful for observation of calcium deposits, configuration of the pulp area, decay, periodontal issues, and other anomalies that are not clinically visible. Advantages of capturing bitewing images is the ease of placement with the sensor in close proximity to the teeth as well as the minimal dimensional distortion that occurs because of the minimal vertical angulations used during this technique. Combinations of periapical and bitewing radiographs are used to take a complete-mouth (CMX) or full-mouth (FMX) x-ray survey.
- There are also **occlusal radiographs** that look at the cutting-edge surfaces of the teeth and the planes in the mouth. Occlusal images can be taken on both the maxillary and mandibular arch. Adult occlusal sensors are captured using size 4 sensors while pediatric occlusal images are captured with size 2 sensors. This type of imaging is useful for observation of obvious abnormalities in the oral cavity as they show large areas of the exposed arch and also allow a 3D view of that area.

PERIAPICAL RADIOGRAPHS
ORIENTATION OF THE PATIENT'S HEAD

Generally, a patient is guided to sit straight and tall during periapical radiography. This position places the plane of the teeth parallel to ground, and the sagittal or right/left midline plane of the head perpendicular to the ground. All points along the ala-tragus line (also known as the maxillary orientation line) should be equidistant from the floor plane for maxillary bone radiographs. The patient's head should be inclined slightly backward during the mandibular shots to rectify the angle changes that occur when the mouth is opened. If muscles on the floor of the mouth become taut, the patient should be instructed to swallow to relax them. Chair height adjustments are often necessary to ensure proper positioning and operator comfort.

PROCEDURAL PARAMETERS FOR PEDIATRIC PATIENTS

The most important consideration when performing radiography on a pediatric patient is the reduction of radiation exposure. This reduction can be optimized by using a longer length positioning device, a rectangular-shaped collimator that fits the shape of the digital sensor, and a beam alignment device that directs the beam to the sensor. In addition, the child's body should be protected by lead shielding using both an apron for the torso region and a cervical collar for the thyroid area. Child seats for positioning are also available

BITEWING RADIOGRAPHS
PROCEDURES FOR THE PREMOLAR AND MOLAR BITEWING RADIOGRAPHS

Size 2 sensors are standard for capturing adult bitewing radiographs. The sensor is placed in the horizontal position in the bitewing RINN XCP and the dental staff must select the bitewing exposure parameters on the control panel of the dental imaging machine. The RINN XCP is held in place by placing it on the hard occlusal surfaces of the bottom teeth and having the patient biting down. The premolar bitewing radiograph is centered in the areas that would be covered by both upper and lower premolar periapical images. The molar bitewing is held similarly and is placed far enough back to cover all three molars. The aiming ring of the RINN XCP is moved into place near the patient's skin, and the exposure is taken.

GUIDELINES FOR VERTICAL AND HORIZONTAL ANGULATION

Most beam alignment devices for bitewings utilize the round shape to match the circular position indicator devices (PIDs) commonly used in dentistry. If the position indicator device is short with an 8-inch distance between the x-ray source and the sensor, it is generally aimed at approximately +10° to the beam alignment device. This is because the sensor tends to angle slightly back from the upper teeth that tilt back, and this vertical angulation establishes a perpendicular relationship between the x-ray beam and the sensor. For a long position indicator device with a source to sensor distance of around 16 inches, the angle can be reduced to 8° for a molar bitewing and 6° for a premolar bitewing. The flat surface of the positioning device should be parallel to the sensor in the beam alignment device. As always, the central portion of the x-ray beam should be aimed at the middle of the sensor.

INSTRUMENTS DESIGNED FOR BITEWING RADIOGRAPHS

Instruments designed for bitewing radiographs typically have a tab or wing connected to the active side of the digital sensor. The tab or wing portion is used for the patient to bite down on which holds the sensor in place during exposure. The tab or wing is positioned on the hard surface of either the molars or premolars (depending on the desired shot) of the lower jaw with the sensor between the teeth and tongue. In order to accomplish this, the technician must initially insert the beam alignment device and sensor by keeping part of the tab against the front of the tooth with one index finger while keeping the sensor portion vertical with the other one. The patient then closes their teeth down on this wing while the operator keeps the tab portion in place. Separate bitewings for the premolar and molar regions using standard size 2 sensor, with the front edges positioned at either the canine or second premolar respectively.

SIZES AND AREAS OF FOCUS

Intraoral dental images can be described in terms of type or area of documentation. The three types come in various sizes for various purposes.

- The first, the periapical image, is used to record the apical or top area of the tooth, nearby bone structures, and crown. This type of image may use a size 0 sensor for children, and sizes 1 or 2 for adult images. comes in a single child size (No. 0) and two adult sizes (No. 1 for the front and No. 2 for the back and bitewings as well).
- Bitewing images are used to document the coronal area and the interproximal alveolar bone crests. These images are captured using the RINN XCP, the most common beam alignment device or by using a bitewing tab or wing and adhering that to the digital sensor and sheath. Both of these methods will allow for the sensor to be stabilized during exposure.
- Occlusal images are much bigger and are designed for use in larger areas like the floor of the mouth or to capture large areas of the maxillary arch. A size 4 sensor is used to capture adult occlusal images and a size 2 sensor is used to capture pediatric occlusal images

FULL MOUTH SERIES

In general dentistry, it is common to expose patients to what is known as a full mouth series. This set of dental images can also be referred to as a full mouth survey or a complete mouth survey. The two types of images that are found in a full mouth series are periapical images and bitewing images.

In a standard adult full mouth series there are 14 periapical images and 4 bitewing images. This allows for the dentist to have a full view of the mouth including all of the teeth in the dentition as well as their surrounding structures and bone. The dental team can adjust the number and types of images found in a full mouth series. Pediatric full mouth series are commonly made of 12 images including 10 periapical images and 2 bitewing images. When exposing an edentulous full mouth series, the dental team will capture the 14 periapical images but will not need the bitewing images as those are used mainly to look for interproximal decay and with an edentulous patient, there are no teeth, and no need for those images. Many digital software systems will allow the dental team to set up an exposure pattern that can be consistently used to capture these images in the same order for each patient. Full mouth series of radiographs are commonly taken every 3-5 years. If a patient is experiencing dental discomfort, the dental team can take individual peripicals and/or bitewings to address that direct need.

OCCLUSAL RADIOGRAPHS
MAXILLARY TOPOGRAPHIC PROJECTION

A maxillary topographic projection is a type of occlusal radiograph designed to document a large portion of the upper jaw. Size 4 sensors and longer 16-inch positioning devices are generally utilized. The smaller potential difference of 65 kVp and 15 mA current are the usual exposure factors. For a maxillary topographic projection, the sensor is positioned in the mouth on the tongue with the active part of the sensor facing upwards towards the maxilla and the inactive part of the sensor down towards the tongue. The dental operator will then ask the patient to bite down gently which will hold the sensor in place. The ala-tragus line should be parallel to the ground, and the midsagittal plane should be at right angle to the ground. The theory of bisecting angles is used to take the x-ray, which means that the central portion of the x-ray beam is directed perpendicular to the bisecting line between the planes of the sensor and the upper incisors. In order to achieve this angulation, the positioning device is usually placed about +65° to the plane of the sensor, near to the nose but not touching it.

MAXILLARY MANDIBULAR CROSS-SECTIONAL PROJECTION

A mandibular cross-sectional projection is a type of occlusal radiograph used to document the presence of anomalies including calcium stones or calcified areas in the salivary glands found in the lower jaw area. Settings are similar to those used for mandibular symphysis projections, but the head is tilted much further back until the plane of the maxillary teeth is actually upright and perpendicular to the floor. The sensor is placed with the active part of the sensor facing downwards towards the tongue and the inactive part facing upwards towards the roof of the mouth. The middle part of the x-ray beam is directed at right angles to the occlusal sensor by positioning the position indicator device close to the lower chin but not touching it.

MANDIBULAR SYMPHYSIS PROJECTION

A mandibular symphysis projection is a type of occlusal radiograph designed to document a large area of the incisor region of the lower jaw. The sensor is placed the same as other mandibular occlusal projections with the active side of the sensor facing downwards towards the tongue. When exposing this projection, the patient's head is inclined backward to form a 45° angle between the floor and the biting surface plane. The midline plane should be perpendicular to the ground. The bisecting angle technique is employed to center the x-ray beam. This translates to an angle between the sensor and x-ray of about 55° and a vertical angulation of about -20°. The beam indicating device is usually placed against the chin.

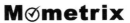

POSTERIOR OCCLUSAL PROJECTIONS

Posterior occlusal topographic projections can be taken for both the upper and lower jaws. For the maxillary jaw, this type of image is useful to view the sinus and other structural areas near the upper dentition. In this case, the sensor is placed lengthwise along the midline on one side of the face, the patient bites down on it, and the positioning device directs the x-ray beam at about a 55° angle through the profile near the premolar region. For the mandible, separate projections for each side of the mouth are usually unnecessary, but if they are required the sensor can again be placed on one side with the long edge positioned anteroposteriorly along the center.

PANORAMIC RADIOGRAPHS

ADVANTAGES

A panoramic radiograph can also be referred to as a pantomogram and is an image that is used to show large areas of the face and oral cavity. These are used when the dental team would like to see more than what the full mouth series or specific periapical or bitewing images can show. In the full-mouth survey, intraoral radiographs show the teeth, alveolar ridges, and some of the associated bone in a specific area of focus. Panoramic tomography extends the observed area far beyond these structures; the jaw, nasal cavities, and temporomandibular joint regions are now included, increasing the diagnostic value. One newer diagnostic use is identification of calcifications in the carotid arteries, which if utilized in conjunction with other tests can help recognize stroke or other cerebrovascular risk. Panoramic techniques are generally easier and less time consuming than intraoral procedures, and therefore tend to cooperate more and have a lower incidence of retakes. With new technology and dental imaging techniques, radiation doses delivered during panoramic techniques are usually less than during other procedures. Panoramic images are also a great alternative for patients who are unable to handle the intraoral full mouth series due to the inability to open their mouth, possible discomfort, or the stimulation of the gag reflex.

DISADVANTAGES

Pantomograms generated during panoramic tomography tend to have a poorer image quality than intraoral radiographs. In particular, the definition is decreased rendering panoramic radiography relatively unsuitable for certain diagnoses. Periodontal disease, tooth decay, and pathological conditions in the periapical region are not picked up well on pantomograms, which means that bitewings and some periapical x-rays used in conjunction may be necessary. Only areas lying within the focal trough or image layer are distinct on panoramic radiographs, and machines with adjustable areas are expensive. In fact, any panoramic machine is generally costly. Lack of clarity can occur due to overlapping of images particularly in the premolar area, superimposition or obscuring of areas especially by the spinal column, and various sources of distortion. The panoramic machine should never be used in cases where only single or limited intraoral radiographs will suffice.

POSTEROANTERIOR PROJECTIONS

A posteroanterior projection is an extraoral exposure of the skull taken by directing the x-ray beam from about 3 feet behind the patient. The central ray is aimed at the occipital protuberance in the ear, with the sensor front of the individual, normally with the forehead and nose positioned against the sensor. This technique is useful for identification of fractures, malignancies, and widespread disease states in the skull area. A variation in which the patient opens their mouth and places their chin and nose against the cassette is called the Waters' view. This change enables visualization of the middle of the face, particularly the maxillary sinus region.

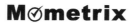

CEPHALOMETRIC RADIOGRAPHS

Cephalometric radiography is a specialized technique that quantifies parameters of the skull in order to predict growth patterns. The method is used primarily by orthodontists or dentists that see mostly children. Cephalometric radiography requires a unique machine that employs an apparatus called a **cephalostat** to hold the individual's head in place with rods and ear posts. All measurements are made relative to the midsagittal or midline plane that divides the face in half, and the Frankfort line is used as the relative horizontal marker. The most popular stance is a lateral exposure with the radiation beam projected a long distance (about 5 feet) from the other side. The radiograph is interpreted by looking at facial relationships and angles in an attempt to predict later growth patterns. Lateral oblique projections, where the beam is at a slight upward angle, are also captured.

CT SCANS

CT or **computed tomography scans** are images produced by directing an x-ray beam at an individual and then digitally transmitting information about the degree of penetration to electronic sensors. The number of pixels in an area is directly related to the density of the tissue, and they are represented as CT numbers or Hounsfield units. Tissue types have characteristic units. For example, water has 0 Hounsfield units, while bone has +1000 units, and air has -1000 units. The beam is projected through the patient while rotating through a plane. This plane can be axial, coronal, or sagittal, meaning it is either parallel to the ground, through the imaginary line dividing the front and back of the head, or through the midline separating right and left. Some CT scanners, in particular those used for the head and neck region, project a beam that is either round or cone-shaped onto a two-dimensional detector. In this case, radiation exposure is minimized.

ADVANTAGES AND DISADVANTAGES

Computed tomography is great at distinguishing between slight differences in tissue density, and in addition contrast and density can be manipulated to look at different areas. CT can be done in a variety of planes while eliminating superimposition of unnecessary images outside the focal plane. Pictures can be reformatted relative to other planes. The technique is easy and accurate. However, the patient is generally exposed to more radiation with CT than with standard imaging techniques, although dosage can be reduced through the use of cone beam machines or software that localizes the imaging. The latter is often used for dental implant preparation. The dental team should be aware that although the CT scanning is a good imaging choice, the same types of errors can occur in this type of imaging as standard dental imaging. This can include any metals in the plane of the image will show up as well as proper positioning. Considerably more radiation is delivered during CT scanning of the head than ordinary skull imaging but this negative aspect is obliterated by the high incidence of repeats in skull imaging. CT scans are more costly to the patient than standard dental images.

CONE-BEAM COMPUTER TOMOGRAPHY (CBCT)

Cone-beam computer tomography takes three-dimensional images through a cone-shaped x-ray beam that moves about the patient's head and face with 360° rotation for 10–40 seconds. While exposing the patient to less x-ray than a standard CT, the dental cone-beam CT still has increased exposure over standard radiography but produces superior images, especially of bony structures and soft tissue, including muscles, lymph nodes, vessels, and nerves. Cone-beam CTs are used primarily in orthodontia. Patients must remove all metal objects on the head and neck as well as removable intraoral prostheses, hearing aids, and underwire bras because the metal may affect the image.

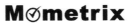

Reviewing Patient Medical and Dental Histories

INDICATIONS FOR RADIOGRAPHIC EVALUATION IN NEW AND RETURNING PATIENTS

If dental history includes any periodontal or endodontic (pulp) treatment, soreness, or evidence of trauma, radiographs will be part of the diagnosis and treatment plan. Radiographs are also commonly taken when there is familial history of dental problems or there is a need to check demineralization or other postoperative conditions including crown placement, implant placement and bone surgery. In addition to familial history and post operative review, there are many other clinically visible signs and symptoms as well as patient complaints that will indicate use of radiographs. These include evidence of various types of dental disease and decay, unexplained symptoms in an area like bleeding, sensitivity, discoloration, and viewing impacted teeth. Sinus problems, neurological abnormalities or asymmetry in the facial region, and temporomandibular joint (TMJ) problems are a few other clinical symptoms that dictate probable use of diagnostic radiography.

UNIQUE SITUATIONS REQUIRING RADIOGRAPHS

Occasionally dental radiographs are taken simply to monitor the growth and development of the oral and maxillofacial region of a child or adolescent. Clinical judgment is necessary in these instances since repeated radiation exposure is involved. Periapical or panoramic images are often taken in adolescents to gauge the development of the third molars. Radiographs can also be done to look at dental implants (or potential sites), assess pathological changes, measure periodontal treatment progress, diagnose dental pulp diseases, locate areas that need restoration, or find minerals in decayed areas.

PATIENT PREPARATION FOR RADIOGRAPHIC EXPOSURE

Patient preparation for radiographic exposure includes:

- **Intraoral radiography**: The patient's head and neck must be examined. The patient must remove glasses and any removable intraoral prosthetics as well as jewelry that lies in the beam path, such as nose and tongue rings/studs. Patient protection includes the thyroid lead collar and lead apron that covers the chest and abdomen.
- **Panoramic radiography**: The patient must remove glasses, removable intraoral prostheses, and hearing aids as well as all head and neck jewelry and metal items, such as earrings, barrettes, and nose and tongue rings/studs. Patient protection includes the panoramic shield apron that covers front and back but is higher in the front than the back because the beam is directed from the back of the head to the front in a superior direction. The thyroid collar is not used because it may interfere with midline imaging. If the apron is longer on one side than the other, the long side should be placed against the patient's back.

ENSURING PROPER COVERAGE FOR X-RAYS

An x-ray should generally include visualization of five tissue types, the tooth enamel, its underlying dentin or hard calcium-containing portion, the sensitive central pulp with nerves and blood vessels, the alveolar or jaw bone, and the surrounding soft tissue. For a periapical image, at least 2 millimeters of bone should be visible around the apices of the teeth that are required for that given image. All areas needed for diagnostic purposes should be included, if possible, with the initial image or visualized on supplemental images such as occlusal image. There are also guidelines for inclusion of other areas like the periodontal membrane space and superimposition of certain cusp tips. Proper coverage can be attained by a combination of the use of a beam alignment device, correct sensor placement, head positioning and radiation settings on the control panel.

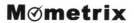

Intraoral and Extraoral Techniques

PARALLELING TECHNIQUES FOR PERIAPICAL RADIOGRAPHS
DECREASING DISTORTION USING SENSOR DISTANCE

Of the two periapical radiographic techniques, the paralleling technique is generally preferred over the bisecting angle technique because there is less distortion. This decrease in distortion is accomplished by the beam alignment device holding the sensor parallel to the long axes of the teeth and directing the beam perpendicular to both. In order to achieve this parallel orientation, the distance between the sensor and the teeth usually needs to be increased, which could theoretically decrease the image clarity. Therefore, sharpness and magnification are usually restored by increasing the distance between the x-ray beam source and the sensor. For this reason, longer 16-inch positioning devices are often utilized. In summary, if you have to increase the distance between the sensor and the teeth, then you must also increase the distance from the position indicator device and the sensor. These combined adjustments will provide the most dimensionally accurate image.

QUANTIFICATION OF THE ANGULATION OF THE X-RAY BEAM

The tubehead of the x-ray machine can be positioned both vertically and horizontally during periapical radiography. The occlusal plane along the top ridge of the teeth should be placed parallel to the floor, and the tubehead height is changed to accommodate this. This **vertical angulation** is calculated in degrees and is positive if the tubehead angles downward or negative if the tubehead angles upward. The angle of the beam is also quantified in terms of its angle from the sagittal plane. In other words, beams directed at back teeth have greater horizontal angles than in the front. This **horizontal angulation** is determined by the location of the targeted teeth. If feasible, the horizontal angle of the beam should also be parallel to the floor and the flat plane of the sensor. The beam should be aimed at the desired area or point of entry, and it should cover the entire sensor and surrounding area to prevent any collimator cutoff.

CRITERIA FOR CORRECT SENSOR PLACEMENT AND POSITION INDICATOR DEVICE POSITIONING

In the paralleling technique, there are six rules for achieving this preferred technique; the first three involve placement of the sensor and the last three cover the positioning of the beam alignment device.

- **Sensor placement**
  - The sensor should be placed in a way that it covers all of the required structures that must be found on that image. If the sensor is not placed properly, this could result in missing teeth and lack of proper diagnosis.
  - The tooth's long axis and the sensors vertical axis should be parallel. Since the apical and occlusal surface of the tooth are both required for periapicals, this rule dictates that the expected distance between the tooth and sensor must often be increased. This increased distance should be used for visualization of teeth in the back of the upper jaw. The front incisors in both jaws tend to tilt outwards, and sensors placed in these areas need to be positioned relatively far back in the oral cavity.
  - The horizontal plane of the sensor should be at the same angle as the mean tangent for the region. The tangent is a flat plane connecting the two end points in the small area being x-rayed.
- **Position Indicator device positioning**
  - The position indicator device should be angled vertically with its flat open end parallel to the sensor container in order to avoid distortion.

25

o The position indicator device should also be angled horizontally to the plane of the area to be covered, thus aiming the x-rays perpendicular to the sensor and the teeth.

o The center of the cone of x-rays must be localized over the middle of the sensor in order to avoid partial images or an incomplete pattern known as cone-cutting or collimator cutoff.

There are different RINN XCP devices for various areas of the mouth and types of projections including anterior periapicals, posterior periapicals, bitewings and endodontic procedures. This is a device that is very technique-sensitive and can be challenging to assemble and set up. To ensure accuracy, the dental team should practice with the RINN XCP prior to actual use on a patient. These also come specific to the different brands of sensors, something the ordering team at the dental office must consider as they purchase the RINN XCP devices and sensors for their office.

IMAGES OF PRE-MOLAR AND MOLAR REGIONS OF THE UPPER ARCH

For the pre-molar and molar regions of the maxillary arch, the beam alignment device is generally used with a size 2 sensor. In these maxillary areas, the alignment device and sensor are placed horizontally to either center the second premolar to capture the premolar region. This will allow for the distal of the canine, the first and second premolar and the first molar to appear on the radiograph. To capture the molar region on an image, the second pre-molar should be lined up with the front edge of the sensor. If the dental assistant is aware that the third molars are impacted or present in the dentition, they should move the sensor slightly further back in the mouth, allowing room to capture the entire third molar... The alignment device is held in place by positioning it against the biting surface of the teeth, inserting a cotton roll below if needed to stabilize it in the mandible, and instructing the patient to bite down to keep it in place. The aiming ring is pulled to touch the patient's skin, and the positioning indicator device is aligned horizontally and vertically before exposure.

IMAGES OF THE ANTERIOR REGION OF THE UPPER ARCH

Images of the front or anterior regions of the maxillary arch are captured using an anterior beam alignment device that holds the sensor in position during exposure. In order to avoid cone-cutting or collimator cutoff, there is a ring that is part of the beam alignment device to allow the dental assistant to know where to place the position indicator device for optimal alignment with the sensor. The dental assistant must ensure that the anterior exposure parameters are set on the x-ray machine. The sensor is centered over a particular tooth depending on the region being radiographed, the maxillary midline for central incisors, the lateral incisor for that region, or the canine for that area. The long axis of the targeted tooth should be parallel to the long axis of the sensor placed in the vertical position. A cotton roll can be placed between the bite block of the alignment device and the teeth in the lower jaw to help stabilize the alignment device and sensor if needed. The aiming ring on the indicator rod is slid towards the patient's skin until it almost touches it, determining the vertical as well as horizontal angulation before the exposure is taken.

PROCEDURES FOR EXPOSURES ON THE LOWER ARCH VS. THE UPPER ARCH

The same beam alignment devices and sensor sizes are used for similar regions in both the maxillary and mandibular arches. The main difference is that the position of the beam alignment device and sensor needs to be inverted or flipped around. For the incisors in the mandible, the biting area of the beam alignment device and the sensor are placed relatively far back near the premolars in order to align the long axis of the teeth in parallel to the sensor, allowing for the most dimensionally accurate image. The biting area of the beam alignment device is centered in much the same manner as for the equivalent area of the maxilla. In the mandibular molar region, the third molar should be covered and the sensor should be placed in the space between the teeth and the

26

tongue. The cotton roll can be placed between the biting area of the beam alignment device and the corresponding maxillary teeth. As in the radiographs for the upper arch, the aiming ring of the beam alignment device is positioned close to the skin, the positioning indicator device is aligned horizontally and vertically, and the exposure is taken.

BISECTING ANGLE RADIOGRAPH TECHNIQUES

CORRECT PLACEMENT AND PROCEDURES

First, the head must be correctly positioned for a bisecting angle radiograph. When capturing images on the maxillary arch, the plane of the teeth being radiographed should be parallel and the midsagittal plane of the head should be perpendicular to the floor. When capturing radiographs on the mandibular arch, the dental assistant should ask the patient to lift their chin slightly which will allow for the occlusal plan of the mandibular teeth to be parallel to the ground. The sensor should be placed in a position where it covers all of the required structures for the image being taken with the middle of the position indicator device being aimed at the center of the sensor. This poisoning will determine the vertical angulation to be used, while the horizontal angulation is determined by directing the beam at right angles to the buccal tangent of the teeth being exposed. The area where the x-ray beam strikes the sensor should be in the center of the sensor. This will prevent cone cutting or collimator cutoff from appearing on the image.

RULE OF ISOMETRY

In order to understand the bisecting technique, it is important to review the rule of isometry. This is because when using the bisecting technique, the x-ray beam is not aimed at a specific structure but one that the dental assistant must conceptualize as they place the sensor and view the oral structures. The rule of isometry asserts that two triangles are equivalent when they have a shared side and two equal angles. What this means in the bisecting angle technique is that the assumption that the central portion of the x-ray beam can be aimed perpendicular to the line that bisects the imaginary angle that is formed between the sensor and the long axis of the tooth (the shared side of the two triangles). In order to visualize this angle, the dental assistant must place the sensor first, and then take a moment to view the sensor in relation to the long axis of the tooth. Then, take that area and divide it in half, and that imaginary angel is where the x-ray beam will be directed. Because the dental assistant is using an imaginary angle to aim the x-ray beam at, distortion will be present because teeth and sensor are not flat planes and are not parallel to each other. It is because of this that the bisecting technique should be used only when the paralleling technique is unable to be achieved. If the position indicator device is angled too low and is close to the angle of the tooth, the image will appear elongated. If the positioning device is angled too high and is close to the angle of the sensor instead, a phenomenon called foreshortening can occur.

VERTICAL ANGULATION OF THE POSITIONING INDICATOR DEVICE

The vertical angulation is the angle between the positioning or beam indicator device and the occlusal plane of the teeth. For the bisecting technique, this angle is always positive for examination of maxillary teeth and usually negative for examinations of the mandibular teeth. The appropriate angle for short 8-inch positioning devices can vary but starting points ranging from +30° for molars and up to +55° for incisors are generally used. The angles are slightly less for longer 16-inch length position indicator devices. When documenting mandibular teeth with this method, the vertical angulation usually ranges from 0° for molars to about -20° for incisors for the short position indicator devices and slightly less for the longer devices. In the past, the dental assistant would have to use their best judgement to determine these angles with both the bisecting and paralleling techniques. In dentistry today, there are many beam alignment devices available to the dental assistant to use and to assist with determining the vertical angulations to be used for each area of the mouth.

27

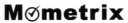

PREVENTING DISTORTIONS IN PARALLELING AND BISECTING TECHNIQUES

MAINTAINING GEOMETRIC SHARPNESS AND MINIMIZING DISTORTION

An image that has a good level of geometric sharpness can be described as one that has clear borders and minimal blurriness., also known as. This is best controlled by the use of an x-ray machine with a small focal spot on the anode target. This is an inherent property of the equipment and cannot be changed and is something that should be considered prior to the purchase of dental imaging equipment. As the distance between the focal spot and the sensor is increased, the sharpness increases. Conversely, as the distance between the object being radiographed and the sensor is increased, the sharpness decreases and more of the resulting image is blurry. These distances primarily affect the magnification of certain areas and their relative distortion. The relationship between true object size and these parameters is as follows:

$$\text{Object size} = \frac{(\text{distance between source and object}) \times (\text{length of image})}{(\text{distance between x-ray source and sensor})}$$

IMPACT OF POSITIONING DEVICES ON MINIMIZING DISTORTION

When possible, the length of position indicator device should be selected based on the technique employed to minimize distortion. The bisecting technique can only be performed with the shorter 8-inch position indicator device generally; it allows the sensor to be positioned close to the teeth to be imaged. Any length device can be used for the paralleling technique since it is placed perpendicular to both the teeth and sensor. The longer tubes (16 inches generally) are better because the distance between focal space and object is increased and sharpness is subsequently augmented.

MINIMIZING DISTORTION CAUSED BY SHAPES AND DIMENSIONS OF OBJECTS

Distortion caused by differences in shape and size can be minimized by two techniques, paralleling and bisecting.

- **Paralleling** refers to the lining the sensor up with the long axis of the tooth that is being imaged so that the tooth and the sensor are in parallel planes and the radiation beam would then be aimed perpendicular to those planes
- **Bisecting** means positioning the radiation beam perpendicular to the midpoint of the angle between the sensor and the long axes of the teeth being radiopgraphed.

Less distortion and greater anatomical accuracy are generally seen with the paralleling technique. In the bisecting technique, the depth dimension differs for various teeth and this can foreshorten or elongate the image.

PANORAMIC RADIOGRAPH TECHNIQUES

ROTATIONAL PANORAMIC RADIOGRAPHY

Rotational panoramic radiography exposes the patient to much less radiation than intraoral procedures; for example, a panoramic view utilizes only about 1/10 the dose of a typical full-mouth survey. It also covers a larger area of the dental arches and surrounding tissues. The images generated by panoramic radiography are comparatively free of distortion and there is little overlay of different structures. Since this is a type of extraoral imaging and there is no manipulation that must occur within the oral cavity, the possibility of disease transmission is greatly reduced. Diagnostically, panoramic radiography offers many advantages, including the decrease in the detection window for decay, periodontal disease, and pulp abnormalities.

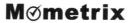

Purpose and Technique

ROTATION OF THE X-RAY

In rotational panoramic radiography, the x-ray beam is rotated in the horizontal plane through a narrow slit around an imperceptible rotational axis in the mouth. The effective focal spot for this plane is essentially the same area targeted on a normal intraoral projection because the moving positions of the ray cross at that position (also identified as the center of rotation). The vertical plane is not influenced by this rotation so its focal spot corresponds to that generated by the x-ray tube. Typically, the vertical plane is angled slightly negative, about -4° to -7°, to direct that aspect through the base of the skull. The extraoral imaging plate is also rotated in the opposite direction through a horizontal axis in order to equilibrate the horizontal and vertical magnifications. Otherwise, the horizontal aspect would be exaggerated relative to the vertical.

TOMOGRAPHY

Tomography is a radiographic procedure that records images in one plane while obscuring or getting rid of images in the other plane. The concept is actually utilized for a number of techniques, including panoramic radiography, computed tomography (CT), and magnetic resonance imaging (MRI). For rotational panoramic radiography, as the x-ray source and imaging plate are rotated around the stationary patient, a tomogram or pantomogram is generated. The unblurred plane is called the focal trough or image layer, and only objects in the center of the intersecting projections will be clear. Therefore, patient positioning is crucial in order to target the desired focal trough.

SEQUENCE OF OPERATION

While there may be some variations with different machines, in general there are five steps involved in patient positioning and subsequent exposure with panoramic radiography:

1. Generally, the first step is to have the patient bite into the groove of the bite block. If the individual is edentulous, a chin rest can be used instead. This step basically centers the patient and their front teeth.
2. Next, guides located on the side of the apparatus are locked in place to steady the patient's head and centralize their rear teeth.
3. The chin is then lowered onto the chin rest, which usually has a slight negative incline equivalent to the upward tilt of the x-ray beam.
4. The cervical spine in the neck is then aligned either by having the individual stand erectly or using any means including pillows to achieve straightening in a sit-down type of machine.
5. The patient is then directed to close their lips and place their tongue against the hard palate and remain still while the technician takes the exposure, which typically lasts up to 22 seconds.

SIX ZONES AND HALLMARKS OF GOOD IMAGES

There are six zones on a panoramic radiograph:

- The largest zone examined on a panoramic radiograph is the **central dentition or array of teeth**. In a good image, each tooth is distinct, the array spreads upward toward the back resembling a smile, the sizes and relative overlap of teeth on both sides are similar, the tops of teeth are not cut off, and front teeth should be clear.
- Above this area is the second zone, or the **nose and sinus region**. Here the lower bones or turbinates of the nasal passage and corresponding air spaces should all appear to be within the nasal cavity, and the hard palate should be observed in this area with the tongue against it. Nasal cartilage should not be visible.
- Below the central dentition is the **mandibular body area**. Not much besides the lower border of the mandible should be observed in this third zone.

- The four corners of the radiograph comprise two different zones. The **upper corners**, Zone 4, should have centered rounded condyles in the temporomandibular joint area. The **lower corners**, Zone 6, should primarily be occupied by the hyoid bone.
- The **areas on the sides** of the center are Zone 5, should show each ramus or branching part of the lower jaw and possibly some of the spine.

POSITIONING LIGHTS

Most panoramic radiographic machines have several positioning lights that are activated before an exposure is taken to ensure correct placement of the patient. Usually there are two vertical lights, one that should be positioned at the corner of the mouth, and another that is focused along the midsagittal plane which should be perpendicular to the floor. There is also a horizontal light that is usually centered along the Frankfort plane, which is the imaginary projection between the floor of the eye socket or orbit and the ear's auditory meatus. In theory, this line should be parallel to the ground. Some panoramic machines have positioning lights that are supposed to run along the ala-tragus instead.

TYPES OF LEAD APRONS

In panoramic radiography, a leaded apron that looks like a poncho covering both the front and the back is used. This can be used to block rays to both the front and back during the rotational pattern of the x-ray beam. However, unlike most other types of exposure, a thyroid collar should not be worn, and the apron should not extend into the thyroid area. The beam in panoramic procedure is angled slightly upward and would be projected into shields in the thyroid region resulting in clear, non-exposed parts on the radiograph. Radiation exposure is not a significant problem, however, because the total dosage used in the panoramic technique is considerably less than with a complete intraoral series.

CONTROLLING THE IMAGE LAYER

There is a direct relationship between the width of the image layer and the effective projection radius. The latter term refers to the distance between the beam's rotational center and the central plane of the image. The relatively unblurred image layer will be increased as this radius increases. The width of the slit beam affects the size of the image layer inversely, so narrow slits augment the size of the focal trough. The speed at which the digital imaging plate is moving also influences the focal trough by modifying the relationship between the rotational center and the focal spot; faster speeds increase the width of the image layer. The x-ray beam is generally moved in a pattern that shifts the effective rotational center along a desired path depending on the area being documented. This requires keeping the central part of the x-ray beam perpendicular to the tangent of the area at each moving point on the curved path.

APPEARANCE OF SOFT TISSUES AND AIR SPACES

It is generally easier to observe soft tissues on panoramic radiographs than with other types of intraoral or extraoral images. This is due to the fact that these types of tissues like cartilage (or fluid) absorb the radiation and thus can appear as light shadows on the x-ray. Nevertheless, poor technique has occurred if structures like the tongue or nose are visible on the image. On the other hand, air spaces do not absorb the radiation and therefore should be black on the radiograph. These characteristic air spaces are known, such as in the nasopharynx, and the presence of other black areas indicates poor methodology as well.

TYPES OF DISTORTIONS

During panoramic radiography, the x-ray beam is always projected slightly downward with some negative angulation. Therefore, teeth or other structures that are closer to the beam and further

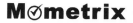

from the digital imaging plate will appear somewhat wider while those that are closer to the imaging plate, which will appear thinner. Additionally, objects toward the back of the oral cavity may appear slightly larger relative to those in the front. Patient positioning can augment these distortions greatly by shifting the focal layer. Only objects in the central plane appear relatively undistorted.

DOUBLE IMAGES

When an anatomical structure or other object is located along the midline, a single image is generated if the entity is between the imaging plate and the rotational center of the radiation beam. However, there is a central diamond-shaped area emanating from the midline where the beam can pick up structures twice as it rotates. Objects in this area can appear on the radiograph as double images. One representation is the mirror image of the other, but both are real. Anatomical structures that often appear as double images include the hard palate and hyoid bone.

GHOST IMAGES

Objects that are situated between the center of rotation and the x-ray source can appear as ghost images on panoramic radiographs. These phantom images are not mirror images. Instead, they show up on the opposing side of the radiograph, relatively blurry, and positioned higher than their real location. The vertical plane of these ghosts is particularly fuzzy because it is magnified more than the horizontal component. Ghost images can often be observed when the object is located relatively posterior to the mandible, either internally like the horn of the hyoid bone or the back of the hard palate, or externally like earrings or other jewelry. Real single, real double, and ghost images can all appear on the same panoramic image.

REMOVAL OF INTRAORAL AND EXTRAORAL ITEMS PRIOR TO PANORAMIC RADIOGRAPHY

If they are not removed, most intra- and extraoral items in the face and neck regions will show up on the panoramic image as both real and ghost images. Any extra oral item has the potential to disrupt the image, and most should be taken off. Artificial hairpieces, non-removable hearing aids, or eye prosthesis are occasionally left in place.

FLATTENING OF STRUCTURES

A panoramic image is generated on a **flat plane**. The midsagittal plane is in the middle of the image but the teeth and other structures on either side are somewhat flattened and spread-out. Structures near to this midline can appear flattened if the patient positioning is incorrect; this is an undesirable condition that may disguise other objects as well.

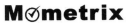

Radiographic Errors and Error Correction

OVERLAPPING MISTAKES

Overlapping on radiographic images can occur as a result of two types of errors. The first type can occur when the flat surface of the sensor is not placed parallel to the front surface or buccal tangent of the teeth being radiographed. As a result, the contacts and openings between the teeth appear to slide over one another or overlap. Incorrect horizontal angulation of the positioning device also can be visualized on a radiograph as overlapping. The most common horizontal angulation error is direction of the beam obliquely, not perpendicularly, to the plane of the sensor. As a result, definition and density are both diminished. Both types of overlapping errors can be corrected by observing the principle of directing the position indicator device perpendicular to the front surface or buccal tangent of the area and keeping the sensor in the same orientation as the teeth.

SENSOR PLACEMENT ERRORS

A common sensor placement error is positioning the sensor too shallow to record the entire tooth while leaving quite a bit of blank area near the crown visible. This error usually occurs because the patient experiences discomfort and does not bite down enough. This is necessary in intraoral imaging as the bite forces the sensor into the area near the apex of the teeth, a required element to be on all periapical images. If the sensor has been placed backwards in the mouth with the inactive surface exposed to the x-ray beam, nothing will be recorded for that image. If the tongue or a finger is in the path of the x-ray beam, it will appear as an artifact on the radiograph. All of these errors warrant repetition of the procedure.

BLANK RADIOGRAPHS AND DENSITY ISSUES

If a radiograph is blank, no radiation was delivered. With digital imaging, this can also present itself as nothing happening on the computer monitor after the exposure button was pushed. Most often this is due to failure to turn on the machine, use the correct tubehead, or properly activating the exposure button. This situation can also occur if the positioning device was severely malpositioned or if a beam alignment device was not used. If the sensor has clearly been exposed, but is very light, the amount of radiation delivered was insufficient for that image or area. A number of factors can influence the quantity of radiation given, therefore when an image appears too light, too dark or no image appears at all, it is a time where the dental assistant must pause and determine what is causing the error.

DISTORTION ERRORS

Distortion of shapes on radiographs results from either improper vertical angulation or incorrect placement of the sensor. Elongation or apparent extension of the tooth image occurs when the vertical angulation used is too small, and the less frequent phenomenon of foreshadowing or apparent reduction of tooth size can happen if the vertical angle used is too large. The relative dimensions of parts of an image can also be distorted when the bisecting angle method is utilized, especially when this technique is applied to documentation of maxillary molars. In this case, the roots are not in the bisecting angle plane and therefore the paralleling method is preferable here.

ERRORS IN PANORAMIC IMAGES
INCORRECT POSITIONING

During panoramic imaging, if the patient bites too far forward into or up against the front of the bite block, the width of the entire image is shrunk. Thus, the most common potential errors are narrowing or missing the crowns of the front teeth or the visible overlap of the cervical spine in the ramus or condyle areas. Sometimes this forward positioning is done intentionally to diagnose sinus

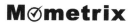

disorders because it also shows the structures in the nasal cavity better. If the patient bites too far back into the groove, the image is widened, which means that all the zones other than the bottom corners are significantly affected. Undesirable visualization of soft tissues can occur, the front teeth are widened, the condyles may be eliminated from view, and ghost images may appear in several areas.

INCORRECT CHIN ANGLE

When the chin is angled downward too much or tipped up too high, the relative curving smile-like configuration of the dentition is changed. An excessive downward chin tilt exaggerates this configuration, while tilting the chin upwards too much destroys this relationship and flattens out the dentition on the image. Consequently, the front teeth of the upper jaw are either quite prominent or their tops are not seen. Front teeth in the lower jaw either have their apices obscured or they are very clear. Sometimes these errors are deliberately exploited to improve the image quality in those areas. In addition, when the chin is tipped too low, the mandible tends to be drawn out vertically in the front and shows images of the hyoid bone, and the condyles may be cut off. If the chin is angled too high, the nasal-sinus cavity can be seen as a large primarily radiopaque area and the condyles may again be eliminated from the image.

ERRORS IF PATIENT'S HEAD IS TILTED IN THE MACHINE

The purpose of closing the side guides on a panoramic machine is to ensure that the individual's head will be upright and not tilted. However, if the patient's head is inclined to the side, this will be very obvious on the radiograph. The back teeth are generally wider and the rows further apart on one side. The mandible looks larger on that side as well, and its lower edge tilts upwards. The condyle on the same aspect also appears to be bigger and higher than the one on the other side. In addition, it is difficult to discern bony details in the upper zones of the image because they tend to be either shadowy or streaked.

ERRORS IF PATIENT IS INCORRECTLY POSITIONED UPRIGHT

The cervical spine in the patient's neck should be straightened before exposing a panoramic radiograph. Sometimes the patient's chin ends up not being against the chin rest. This does not affect the documentation on the central dentition area of the radiograph, but structures normally on the top third of the x-ray are cut off, and little is seen on the bottom third. If the individual is slumped over and the spine is not straight, a ghost image of the spine tends to obscure other structures, primarily the front teeth in the central dentition zone as well as parts of the lower jaw.

ERRORS IN THE EXPOSURE STEP

During the exposure step of panoramic radiography, there are generally three kinds of errors that might occur.

- If the patient does not close their lips and place their tongue against the palate as directed, air between the lips masks the crowns of the front teeth and another air space in the palatoglossal region between the tongue and palates obscures the apices and bone in the maxillary jaw.
- If the patient moves during the exposure, the main radiographic errors observed are waves or other distortions in the mandible.
- Mistakes in the actual exposure process can also be made with images being either too light or too dark, a common indicator of an incorrect exposure setting.

33

Purpose and Technique

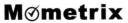

PROCEDURAL ERRORS

One common procedural error in panoramic radiography is beginning at the wrong place during exposure. This results in loss of part of the anatomic region desired, which shows up on the radiograph as a blank area. Another procedural mistake is failure to remove thick clothing, to place the lead apron correctly, or to adjust for individuals with short necks or broad shoulders. In this case, as the cassette rotates around it may find resistance when it touches the individual. When this disengagement occurs, a vertical band of the imaging plate will be overexposed and darker compared to the rest of the image. Some dental offices take out the bite block or other parts (a practice that is discouraged), which can cause a number of radiographic errors including lack of clear separation between rows of teeth and mispositioning of the patient.

RADIOGRAPHIC CHALLENGES ASSOCIATED WITH ENDODONTICS

Endodontic radiography is primarily used to look for dental pulp diseases. When capturing intraoral periapical images in endodctic dentistry, the sensor is held in place by an endodontic beam alignment device, These endodontic beam alignment devices are made in such a way that they inherently allow for extra room in the biting area to account for files and other endodontic materials that may be inside the pulp chamber during imaging. Usually, several different views are necessary to get a three-dimensional perspective. When the endodontic beam alignment device will not allow for proper sensor placement, a hemostat may work to hold the sensor in place, especially in the molar and pre-molar regions of the lower jaw. A number of views are usually documented, including from the top, from the back, and from the side.

CORRECTION OF ERRORS IN ACQUIRED IMAGES

The following errors in acquiring images can be corrected by:

- **Distortion**: Switch from the bisecting angle to a parallel angle for intraoral images as this increases clarity and reduces distortion.
- **Contact surface overlap**: Correct horizontal angulation or beam alignment devices placement. Correction should be made if the overlap includes more than 50% of the enamel width.
- **Shortened images**: Result from excessive vertical angulation. Decrease angulation by 10° or more.
- **Lengthened images**: Results from insufficient vertical angulation. Increase angulation by 10° or more.
- **Off-centering of occlusal plane with bitewings**: Correct placement of the sensor by centering the beam alignment device on the tooth and first seating distal part before moving medially.
- **Crowns of anterior teeth missing**: Results from excessive vertical angulation for bisecting angle or incorrect sensor position for parallel angle. For bisecting, decrease the vertical angulation. For parallel, reposition beam alignment device and sensor.
- **Apices missing**: Increase vertical angulation. Switching from bisecting to parallel view may alleviate problem.
- **Cone-cutting**: Results from incomplete coverage of the sensor by the position indicator device. Reposition the position indicator device over the sensor and verify coverage before exposure.
- **Blurred image**: Results from movement of some type. Remind patient to hold very still.

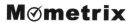

TYPES OF MODIFICATIONS POSSIBLE IN DIGITAL IMAGING

Various software and other tools incorporated into digital imaging processing equipment can be used to modify the image for better visualization or diagnostic purposes. One of the most common software packages can turn over the generated picture to give the mirror image; this is used to orient the views like a set of conventional images. There are various controls that can change the brightness, manipulate the contrast into a suitable gray scale range, or zoom for magnification of specific areas. There is usually a mechanism to exchange black and white areas or reverse the gray scale in order to see certain objects better, and another that colorizes or designates a color to the gray ratio. The computer usually has incorporated filters to reduce noise and sharpen the picture. Software may also permit measurement of certain areas on the image.

SUBTRACTION RADIOGRAPHY

Subtraction radiography is a technique employed with digital image processing. The technique digitally merges two different images and then subtracts the common areas from the radiographic representation. Therefore, only the variations between the original images are seen. This practice is useful for visualization of sequential changes in decay development or bone loss as well as for observation after surgical procedures such as implants or periodontia. At present, the legal implications of permanent storage of this type of manipulation of the images as well as other modifications are somewhat unresolved. Usually, the manipulated image can only be earmarked as a copy, not an original.

Radiographic Equipment Utilized in Digital Imaging

BASIC EQUIPMENT

With the transition from traditional film based imaging to digital imaging in dentistry came the need to utilize current x-ray equipment differently and to purchase new equipment to allow for the acquiring and viewing of digital images. The dental x-ray machines that create the radiation used to capture images were able to be calibrated to make the transition from film based imaging to digital imaging. With current technology, calibration technicians are able to determine what amount of radiation the same machines need to produce for the digital sensors. As an advantage, this amount is typically 60-90% less than the amount of radiation needed for film based images. Dental teams are trained on how to adjust the machines and where to look for the radiation levels for the various projections utilized in their offices.

The components on the x-ray machines including the tubehead. extension arm, and control panel are adjustable. The dental assistant will manipulate the tubehead and the extension arm for every image they take. The tubehead is the device that is connected to the position indicator device and is what is used to position the x-ray beam prior to exposure. The extension arm is what connects the tubehead to the control panel and also is what contains the electrical cords from the outlet to the tubehead, essential in creating the radiation to take the images. The control panel is where the settings that determine how much radiation is created and how fast that radiation will travel. This is changed when images are exposed in various areas of the mouth including anterior posterior and when bitewings are captured. This is due to the varying levels of bone, with some areas of the mouth have thicker bone and need more radiation and others have less and need limited radiation exposure. The control panel and the tubehead will not release any radiation until the exposure button is pressed. Typically, this is on a flexible cord that allows the dental assistant to move to a safe position or can be built into the wall outside of the dental operatory. In both cases, the dental assistant must be able to physically view the patient during the full exposure in the event that the digital sensor needs repositioning.

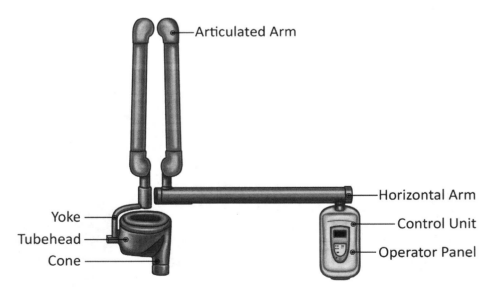

The control panel controls how much radiation is created within the dental tubehead. When the x-ray machine is plugged into an electrical outlet and turned on, based on the setting, radiation will automatically begin to form in the dental tubehead. This happens through a number of different

Purpose and Technique

components. The step up transformer is the component in the tubehead that takes the electrical energy from the wall outlet and turns it into the amount that is needed by the tubehead to create radiation. It is a significant increase from standard electrical input, with increases from the standard 110 or 220 volts to over 3000 volts of energy. This energy goes from the wall to the filament circuit on the cathode side or the negatively charged side of the tubehead , which then heats up due to the large amount of energy. Through this heating, a process known as thermionic emission occurs, and electrons are created. These electrons sit in a cloud and wait for the exposure button to be activated. When the exposure button is activated, the electrons will move at a very high rate of speed from the tungsten filament to the tungsten target. They will collide with the tungsten target and due to the force of that collision, the electrons will transform into radiation. The tungsten target is built into anode side of the tubehead, or the positively charged side at an angle. This allows for the radiation beams that are created to be directed outside of the tubehead to the patients area of concern. To filter the beam and ensure that medically beneficial beams come into contact with the patient, the x-rays go through a collimator to help shape the size of the beam that strikes the patient as well as what are known as aluminum disks. These disks create a filter that removes any beams that are moving too slowly or are not helpful in the capturing of the area being imaged.

Dental X-Ray Tube

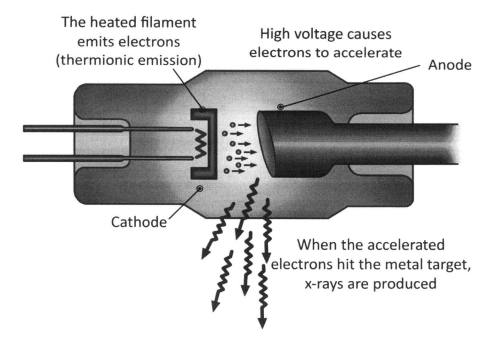

Along with the x-ray machine, the dental team will need to have computer equipment in each operatory where digital images will be captured including a monitor, computer base, keyboard, and mouse. This will allow for the digital sensor to deliver the latent image from the sensor to the computer system, where it can be processed or digitized for viewing.

DIGITIZATION

Digitization is the transformation of pieces of an analog image into relative intensities and the reassembly of these intensities into a visible image on a computer screen. An ordinary radiograph is

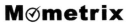

an analog image because the finished product is a direct representation of what has been documented on film. Digital procedures take the analog image and initially convert it to numbers on a grid that represent relative levels of brightness. The number within each grid measures the number of pixels in that area. No film or processing is required with digital imaging and the radiation dose is up to 90% less than that of conventional film based dental radiography. The computer-generated images can be viewed right away, manipulated, or transmitted electronically.

DIGITAL IMAGING RECEPTORS

Traditional film based radiography has been replaced with digital radiography. That means that not only is a computer system used to show the resulting image but the device used to receive the radiation and the latent image has changed too. Today, a direct or indirect digital sensor is used in place of traditional film. These sensors can be different sizes than traditional film was to allow for placement in various areas of the oral cavity. Size 0 are commonly used for pediatric patients, size 1 for narrow adult anterior images, size 2 is the standard adult size and the occlusal size for pediatric patients and size 4 is the adult occlusal size sensor. They can be made of ridged plastic and connected to a cord, an example of a direct digital sensor, or they can be made of a softer bendable type of material without a cord that attaches the sensor or receptor to the computer. Both types are made of materials that capture the image, but in an electronic manner and converts the radiation received into an image that will appear on the computer screen.

The dental team must be intentional about selecting the type of digital sensor they would like for use in their office. Some have sharper corners and some have smoother corners, some are thicker and can be more of a challenge to place in the oral cavity and some are easier to place. The dental team must learn to care properly for the digital sensors, as each direct sensor that is wired with a cord can cost upwards of $12,000. These can also be damaged during patient use; therefore, the dental team must be able to guide the patient on how to properly bite with the digital sensor in place. Manufacturers have also made numerous beam alignment devices that fit these sensors, many which are brand-specific and again, have different advantages. There are two main types of digital receptors, the first being the charge-coupled device (CCD), which may be wired or wireless, but the sensor is bulkier and inflexible. The other type is the photostimulable phosphor plate (PSP), which is flexible and similar to film but is reusable.

THE USE OF BEAM ALIGNMENT DEVICES IN DIGITAL INTRAORAL IMAGING

Digital imaging utilizes different types of beam alignment devices than conventional films. These devices have been manufactured in a way that, when used with digital sensors, proper sensor placement, and correct position indicator alignment, dimensionally accurate images will be produced. In the past, these were referenced as film holding devices, stabes, bitewing tabs, hemostats or snap-a-rays. While some of these have been completed replaced by the beam alignment devices, others have been altered so that they can be used with both direct and indirect digital sensors. The most common beam alignment device in digital imaging is the RINN XCP. This is a device that is made of a strong plastic bite tab, a metal rod, and a strong circular or rectangular ring. When assembled correctly, there will be the circular ring at one end, connected to the strong plastic bite tab at the opposite end. The dental assistant will place the sensor onto the plastic bite tab into a notch that exists for the sensor. That part of the beam alignment device will then be placed into the correct location in the oral cavity. Once positioned, the dental assistant will move the plastic ring towards the face until it is almost touching the patients face. They will finalize the procedure by lining up the circular position indicator device with the plastic ring. Once stabilized the image will be exposed and reviewed.

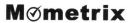

DIGITAL IMAGING SENSORS

CHARGE COUPLED DEVICE

A charge coupled device or CCD is one type of sensor that can detect x-rays and transform them into electronic data for computer interpretation and visualization. CCDs consist of transistor grids that change x-ray photons striking them into electrons. CCDs can be used with visible light. For x-ray exposures, the beam passes through a scintillation screen and a fiber-optic faceplate before reaching the CCD sensor. The scintillation screen serves to convert the x-ray picture into fluorescing visible light. The fiber-optic plate focuses the light and reduces passage of the x-rays by use of leaded glass. The CCD receives the light as pixels on the grid, which are then interpreted in terms of brightness and position to form a digital image. CCDs are used in direct digital imaging or indirectly in conjunction with a scanner.

CMOS/APS

CMOS/APS is the abbreviation for a Complementary Metal Oxide Semiconductor with an Active Pixel Sensor. It is another device used to directly produce digital images from x-ray exposure. It is similar to a CCD in that it employs a scintillation screen to convert the x-rays to visible light and an integrated circuit board to convert the light to digital images for computer interpretation. The main difference between CMOS/APS devices and CCDs is that the CMOS/APS includes amplifying transistors on each of the pixels. Advantages of CMOS/APS sensors include the ability to put circuitry directly onto the chip, use of less power, and reduction of pixel size. These devices can also be linked to a computer via a simple USB port.

DIGITAL IMAGING WITH CMOS OR CCD SENSORS

Detectors used for CMOS or CCD digital imaging are thicker than the conventional film that was used in dentistry in the past, therefore it can be more challenging to place and harder for the patient to tolerate. This difference means that beam alignment devices must be utilized to assist in the placement of the CMOS or CCD sensors. After positioning, the software in the computer regulates the sensor and clarifies the appropriate time to snap the exposure. Since no development is necessary for either of these techniques, the image is available within seconds, and the viewpoint or characteristics of the picture can be modified with the software. Digital imaging that uses these CMOS or CCD sensors is known as direct digital imaging. It is called direct digital imaging because the wired sensor that is connected to the computer goes into the patient's mouth. Following the exposure to radiation, the image appears directly from the sensor onto the computer screen; there is nothing that the dental assistant must do to make that process occur. Because of this speed and convenience, direct digital imaging is the preferred method for most dental offices.

ACQUIRING DIGITAL IMAGES DIRECTLY WITH PSP IMAGING

Photostimulable phosphor (PSP) imaging is one method of converting x-ray exposures directly into digital images. Rare earth phosphors, typically barium europium fluorohalide, are coated onto imaging plates. When x-rays strike these plates, the radiation energy is amassed on the plate as a type of latent image until processed by a PSP scanning machine. Following the exposure of a set of images with the PSP plates, they are scanned into the computer system with a laser to produce fluorescence. The signals are interpreted by a photodiode which transfers the digital image to a computer. PSP imaging uses PSP plates that are available in the same size as the CMOS or CCD sensors, but allow for more flexibility in the placement of the PSP plates. Other advantages of this system include less radiation to the patient, an expanded and linear range of exposures that can produce a good image, and the ability to take an image without being hooked up to a computer. This type of digital imaging that uses these PSP plates is referred to as indirect digital imaging, as the dental assistant will expose the PSP plate to radiation, but must wait and perform an intermediary

39

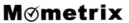

step of scanning in the PSP plate before the image will appear on the screen. These sensors do allow for some bending and flexibility; because of this they are commonly used in pediatric offices where the patients oral cavity is much smaller and more challenging to fit digital sensors into comfortably.

STEPS INVOLVED IN PSP DIGITAL IMAGING

For digital imaging that utilizes photostimulable phosphors, the first step is the erasure of images on the plates from previous exposures. This step is very easy. Basically, the phosphor-coated side of the plate is set on top of a lighted viewbox for several minutes to obliterate the prior image. Then the plates are enclosed in tight barrier envelopes or the panoramic cassette. The x-ray exposure is taken. Then the covering is removed, and the PSPs are loaded onto a drum. This drum is placed into the scanner, and the exposures are scanned with a laser. The images are transmitted directly to a computer where the dental assistant can organize them into the desired viewing order.

ADAPTING DIGITAL IMAGING FOR PANORAMIC OR CEPHALOMETRIC MACHINERY

When capturing images utilizing the panoramic or cephalometric machines with PSP or CCD technology compared to intraoral images there are a few adaptations to be aware of. The size of the digital plate or sensor that receives the image is much smaller for intraoral images than it is for panoramic or cephalometric, as are the PSP or CCD scanners used to transfer the image from the sensor to the computer system. Another important difference to understand is resolution of the panoramic or cephalometric image and how it is affected by the use of the PSP system or the CCD system. When using the PSP technology for panoramic images, the exposure time can be greatly reduced as well as the resolution of the image due to a reduction in line pairs per millimeter on the sensor. With the CCD technology, there is minimal resolution reduction, meaning that the line pairs per millimeter is not affected as it is with the PSP technology and the resolution of the resulting image is not affected. This is one advantage of using the CCD technology over the PSP technology for panoramic and cephalometric imaging. The machines that use CCD technology use multiple CCDs stacked into a grid-like linear array. The array travels around or scans the individual gathering a series of single vertical lines to form the image.

HOW DIRECT DIGITAL IMAGE SENSORS INTERFACE WITH THE COMPUTER

CCDs currently interface with the computer for digital imaging via a Universal Serial Bus (USB) or Firewall connector. Older CCD sensor systems utilize computers with special circuit boards incorporated into them, but newer models can process the picture through external packs or processing boards. CMOS/APS sensors generally interface with the computer through a simple USB port. Both CCD and CMOS sensors produce images on the computer within seconds. PSP plates do not directly connect to the computer; instead, the laser scanner (which fluoresces the latent image on the plate) is directly attached to the computer. The time between exposure and reading for PSP imaging is much longer than that required with the other sensors.

STORING DIGITAL RADIOGRAPHIC IMAGES

Original or manipulated images can be stored on the computer with software that typically compresses or reduces the size of the file. Files can be compressed with either no loss of computer data or with some ("lossy") deficit of original data. Both methods permanently change the image, but studies have found that diagnostic utility is not compromised with compression up to 1/12 of the original. Digital image formats include TIFF, which does not discard any data, and JPEG, which does reduce the image as much as 100 times and is therefore a lossy compression. Thus, the JPEG format can initiate image degradation. Typically, the images are also backed up on DVDs or other storage media. They can also be transmitted via networking to other individuals.

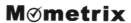

SELECTION OF COMPUTER AND OTHER COMPONENTS OF DIGITAL IMAGING

When selecting a computer to perform digital imaging, either a laptop or desktop model can be used. The processor speed determines the rapidity of image processing. Sufficient RAM should be chosen to enable data retention and processing during the exposure without having to temporarily store the information on the hard drive. After processing, the image probably will be kept on the hard drive so its memory should be large. Various types of printers, each with its own pros and cons, can be selected. A number of dental imaging software packages are available; it is preferable to buy one that conforms to standards established by Digital Imaging and Communications in Medicine (DICOM).

QUALITY ASSURANCE OF RADIOGRAPHIC EQUIPMENT

Quality assurance is the summation of administrative and technical steps required to maintain reliable and reproducible results in any type of work setting. In the context of a dental radiological setup, quality assurance efforts translate to practices that will assure consistent, comprehensible radiographs with minimal radiation exposure. There are usually two components to quality assurance. The first component is quality administration, which is the administrative aspect of coordinating efforts to ensure high-quality work. The other part to quality assurance is quality control, which encompasses the actual test procedures and technical practices required to maintain consistent, first-rate results.

RECOMMENDED QUALITY CONTROL PRACTICES

Auxiliary equipment such as leaded aprons, thyroid jackets, digital sensors and the x-ray tubehead and control panel need to be checked at regular intervals. In addition to standard documentation logs, documentation should also include a retake log book of images taken by the dental team that needed to be retaken due to being of poor quality, which includes explanations of errors for reference and a general quality assurance register that records all procedures, outcomes, and remedial actions taken. Settings for exposure parameters under all possible scenarios should be clearly displayed in the work area. All equipment measurements and manuals should be readily available.

CHECKING X-RAY MACHINE'S POTENTIAL DIFFERENCE AND ACCURACY

The potential difference or kVp, the precision of its setting, and the size of the focal spot all influence the quality of the x-ray beam emitted from the machine. These parameters should be checked once a year. The test generally used to evaluate the potential difference or penetrating power of the beam is the half-value layer test. Sheets of aluminum of various thicknesses are placed between the positioning device and a pocket dosimeter. With the x-ray equipment at highest voltage or potential difference, the beam is directed through the aluminum and the output in mR is measured by the dosimeter. Half of the maximal output should pass through a particular disc as outlined by federal guidelines; failure to do so indicates needed repair.

Accuracy of the voltage setting is typically checked with commercially available meters. These meters quantify the wavelength and frequency of a beam directed at a target; since potential difference determines these two parameters, its accuracy is ascertained.

USE OF POCKET DOSIMETER IN QUALITY CONTROL

A pocket dosimeter is a small rod-shaped ionization chamber used to quantify the radiation being emitted from the x-ray machine. It basically consists of an air-filled chamber, a quartz fiber, a lens, and a switch that is charged prior to use. The dosimeter is used to compare radiation produced through a series of exposure settings relative to the same settings at baseline. The number of milliroentgens generated or the relative gray scale on a wedge should be equivalent to the baseline

41

values. If the current readings do not match the reference value, then the timer and the mA circuit must be checked as well. There are commercially available meters to check timers, but this can also be done manually by directing the central x-ray beam perpendicularly to a spinning top apparatus attached to a sensor and counting the number of dots shown on the sensor. After checking the timer, the filament or mA circuit can be evaluated in one of two ways. If more than one current setting is available, output in milliroentgens can be measured at the same theoretical mAs product for each; if readings do not match, repair is indicated. With only one mA setting available, outside servicing is required. These procedures should be performed yearly.

CHECKING AND EVALUATING THE FOCAL SPOT SIZE

The focal spot size is the surface area covered by the x-ray beam. Typically, the spot size deteriorates and becomes larger over time due to constant bombardment with electrons. If the spot size is enlarged, the resolution or ability to differentiate adjoining structures in the image is decreased. Spot size is checked with a simple plastic tube, usually 6 inches in length. The tube has a leaded closed end with slots that the position indicator device is placed against, and an open end that is positioned over a size 4 occlusal sensor. Exposure is performed, and the resolution on the resulting test image is evaluated by counting the number of line pairs per millimeter that can be resolved. Generally, if the resolution is less than or equal to 7 pairs per millimeter, resolution is inadequate. In this case, either a new machine should be bought, or the tubehead can be reconstructed.

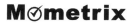

Patient Management

MANAGING PAIN AND ANXIETY

Some patients are anxious or tend to experience discomfort during radiography. If all desired areas can be visualized on a panoramic radiograph, its substitution for intraoral procedures can alleviate anxiety and discomfort. If an intraoral sensor must be used on a patient with anxiety, there are ways to relax the muscles in the area being x-rayed and help ease the patients worries. These include placing the sensor closer to the tongue or using commercially available tissue pads attached to the top edge of the sensor sheath, which will prevent it from sticking directly to the sensor. Anesthetics can be applied topically to the region, but they should be rinsed out after the dental procedures. Occasionally, patients are given prescription tranquilizers like diazepam to reduce their apprehension.

MANAGING PATIENTS WITH SPECIAL NEEDS

A good chairside manner is paramount in dealing with any patient. The major physical disability that might pose a problem in dental radiology is a patient's **inability to control movement** as in certain spastic disorders; here a friend wearing protective gear should assist and steady the patient, not the dental professional. Individuals with **developmental disabilities** are usually harder to manage, and use of sedatives or anesthesia may be necessary. Most types of radiographs can be done without moving an immobile patient out of a wheelchair, and if they are confined to their beds or home, there are mobile x-ray units available. Alternative methods of communication need to be used with individuals who have **hearing or vision impairment**.

MANAGING PEDIATRIC PATIENTS

Pediatric patients may be unfamiliar with the process of having x-rays taken, so any attempt to explain or show them what will occur during the exposure is helpful. One of the major management issues is getting the pediatric patient to understand that they must remain perfectly still when the shot is being taken. In addition, some children cannot endure certain types of intraoral sensor placements. Since their mouth is smaller than that of an adult, more latitude can be allowed in the technique or placement of the sensor. For example, an acceptable exposure can be taken by having the child bite down on a periapical sensor beam alignment device while the operator increases the vertical angulation. Reverse bitewings are often done on pediatric patients because they tend to dislodge regular bitewings; in the reverse technique the bitewing is positioned near the cheek and the exposure is taken as a lateral oblique view from the opposite side. Occasionally, extraoral images such as a panoramic are done instead.

GAG REFLEX

The gag reflex is the tendency to choke or vomit. A portion of dental patients will experience this tendency during dental procedures such as radiography. The reflex is initiated when its receptors, which are located on the back third of the tongue as well as the rear of the throat, are irritated. Nerves located in these regions send messages to the gag center in the medulla oblongata portion of the brain. Nerves from the brain transmit signals to muscle fibers associated with the gag reflex. Initially, the patient cannot breathe, and later muscles in the upper part of the abdominal cavity and the upper portion of the throat contract. This choking reaction may be accompanied by regurgitation of undigested food as well.

INTERVENTIONS FOR PATIENTS WITH A SEVERE GAG REFLEX

Interventions for severe gag reflex include the following:

- Have the patient breathe through the nose.
- Have the patient breathe slowly and concentrate of breathing.
- Spray the back of the patient's throat with an anesthetic mouth spray, such as Chloraseptic.
- Have the patient make a tight fist with the left hand and concentrate on it.
- Rinse the patient's mouth with salt water before examination.
- Talk to and distract the patient.
- Ask the patient to lean forward when taking impressions so material doesn't ooze toward the back of the throat.

RESULTS OF POOR PATIENT PREPARATION

Patient preparation errors with regard to unacceptable radiographic images generally fall into two categories.

- The first category is the additional **overlapping of radiopaque artifacts**. These artifacts result from failure to remove primarily metallic hardware from the body or oral cavity. Examples include dental hardware, many types of jewelry, glasses, and artificial hairpieces.
- Any type of movement from the patient including touching the equipment can result in **unsharpness or blurring** of the image by increasing the peripheral penumbra area of the focal spot.

Good chairside technique from the technician should eliminate these errors.

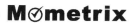

Digital Image Mounting

ARRANGING A FULL MOUTH SURVEY

When exposing images using the direct or indirect digital technique, the images do appear on a computer screen, but it does not mean they will always appear in the correct location. This means that the dental assistant must know the proper placement for each image and must also know how to utilize the computer system to move the images around if needed. Typically, in a full mouth survey, the back teeth of the upper jaw are arranged first with their crowns facing downwards, using landmarks of the dental arch to distinguish pre-molars from molars. Then maxillary teeth toward the front are arranged with their edges facing downward. The incisors are placed in the center with laterals and canines to the appropriate side as identified by landmarks. Similarly, mandibular radiographs are arranged with the crowns or incisal surfaces facing upwards. Bitewing images are found in the center of a digital mounts as they contain the crowns for both the upper and the lower teeth. The premolar bitewing images will be in the center of the mount with the molar bitewing images being in the outer portion of the mounting platform. A useful landmark for these radiographs is the root pattern, as molars in the lower jaw have two roots while those in the upper jaw have three.

TYPICAL ANGULAR CONFIGURATION OF TEETH

In the upper jaw or maxilla, most teeth are angled outward from the jaw. This configuration is known a buccal or facial tilt. In the lower jaw or mandible, the angle between the teeth and the jaw typically changes from a buccal tilt in the front six teeth to an almost upright orientation at the premolars to a small inward or lingual tilt at the back. The real axis of the root of a tooth is the line between the tip of the root, which is not visible to the eye, and the end of the visible part of the tooth. Assumptions about the location of the tip or apical area of the root in the maxilla can be made by envisioning a line between the tragus, the bulge anterior to the ear opening, and the ala or wing of the nose and extrapolating to identifying facial features. The line for similar extrapolation to the mandible is about a half centimeter below the jaw.

Purpose and Technique

45

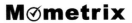

Image Viewing

DIFFERENTIAL ABSORPTION OF X-RAYS

Tissues and other materials found in the jaw area are subject to differential absorption of x-rays. Metals used in restorations tend to have high atomic numbers and thus absorb a greater proportion of x-rays. Therefore, restorations and to a lesser extent enamel and cortical bone usually are observed on dental images as radiopaque areas. This means that those areas are very bright and transparent because they have already absorbed the x-ray energy and it does not strike the sensor located behind the structure being radiographed. At the other end of the spectrum, dark or radiolucent portions of the radiograph result from areas that are easily penetrated by the x-ray. These include the softer tissues. Scattering can produce similar dark spots. Teeth and bones are comprised of a considerable amount of calcium and phosphorus, but the rate of absorption can be affected by age and presence of decay or other disease in these structures.

INTERPRETING STRUCTURES ON RADIOGRAPHS

Teeth and other structures or areas on a radiograph are generally interpreted in terms of how radiolucent or radiopaque they are. Radiolucent areas allow a great deal of radiation to penetrate them and thus appear dark or black on the radiograph. Radiopaque areas block the passage of x-rays and thus emerge as relatively light or white on the radiographic image. Radiopaque sections are described as being denser than radiolucent portions. These known density differences are used to interpret the structures and processes observed on the radiograph or a computer-generated image.

AREAS OF MOUTH THAT ARE RADIOLUCENT

There is a cavity enclosed by the dentin and enamel of the tooth called the pulp space. This cavity is radiolucent or dark on a radiograph generally. The portion protruding down into the apex of the root of the tooth is termed the root canal space, and it should appear radiolucent on the image as well. The pulp areas can become inflamed secondary to microbial infections from injury or diseases of the teeth or surrounding areas. Typically, there is also a dark or radiolucent border between the lamina dura and the root section of the teeth representing the periodontal ligament space (PDLS). This space appears wider in a number of metastatic diseases or if the teeth have been shifted (primarily through orthodontia).

AREAS OF MOUTH THAT ARE RADIOPAQUE

The enamel of the teeth, the dentin underneath, and another part called the lamina dura all appear as white or somewhat light areas (radiopaque) on a radiograph. These structures all absorb the x-rays to some extent. The enamel or hard calcium-containing layer on the outside of the tooth is very white on a radiograph, while the underlying dentin is slightly less dense and appears lighter on the image. Tooth decay or caries can be visualized in both these areas. There is also a very delicate layer of alveolar bone surrounding the tooth socket called the lamina dura which also should be radiopaque on the radiograph. This bone becomes thicker at the top when a new tooth is emerging, and it can shrivel or disappear in certain disease states. The other portions of the alveolar bone surround the teeth and are relatively radiopaque as well. Thinning of this bone suggests a disease state such as periodontal disease or even osteoporosis.

STRUCTURES IN MAXILLA THAT APPEAR RADIOLUCENT

The anatomical structures of the maxilla or upper jaw that appear radiolucent on a radiograph are those that are some type of natural opening or groove. One of these structures is the median maxillary or palatal suture. This structure is a fixed joint in the roof of the mouth beginning at the center of the incisors and extending posterior along the midline. There is also a dark cavity to either

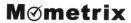

side of the front of this line called the nasopalatine or incisive foramen, whose major function is to receive nerve responses and blood vessels. Occasionally, four cavities are observed instead of two. If the area has a white border, cyst formation is suggested. Any hollows containing air are dark-appearing nasal fossae, including small indentations in the alveolar bone of either jaw called incisive lateral fossae. These areas do not indicate disease processes. Parts of the maxillary sinus appear radiolucent as well.

STRUCTURES IN THE MAXILLA THAT APPEAR RADIOPAQUE

There are several characteristic anatomical structures in the maxilla that appear radiopaque or relatively white on a radiograph. Typically, a white section that looks like an inverted Y is seen in the canine area. This inverted Y represents the junction between the front border of the maxillary sinus and the floor of the nasal fossa. This area is used as a landmark even in toothless individuals, and pathological conditions can change its appearance. Tuberosities are rounded protuberances found in the back of the jaw; they also are relatively radiopaque. Just behind the tuberosity is another light area that resembles a hook, called the hamular process. One of the cheek bones in the upper jaw is termed the zygomatic or malar bone, and it is generally visualized as a radiopaque U-shaped area or arch above the teeth.

STRUCTURES IN THE MANDIBLE THAT APPEAR RADIOLUCENT

In the front of the mandible, there are two radiolucent areas. The first is the mental foramen, which is a round-shaped section just below both sets of pre-molars; its serves as a tributary for nerve impulses and blood vessels. There is a genial tubercle along the midline in the front of mandible, which appears as a dark spot in the middle for passage of blood vessels surrounded by a lighter area where muscles are attached. There is also a dark passage called the mandibular or inferior alveolar canal that runs down the side of the lower jaw between the mandibular foramen and the mental foramen. A major artery traces the canal area and relatively light areas are seen to either side.

STRUCTURES IN THE MANDIBLE THAT APPEAR RADIOPAQUE

The coronoid process is the forward-sloping triangular shaped portion of the mandible or lower jaw. It projects from the sigmoid notch of the mandible and connects to a muscle called the temporalis. This process appears relatively radiopaque on a radiograph, and it is often seen on images of the maxilla because of its proximity. Other radiopaque areas in the front of the mandible include the mental ridges or bones on the front of the lower jaw, parts of the genial tubercles below and along the midline, and the lower cortex of the jaw. White lines are also seen extending from the mental tubercle back to the anterior portion of the branching ramus (the external oblique ridge) and lingually from the pre-molar to molar regions (mylohyoid line).

APPEARANCE OF MAXILLARY SINUS ON RADIOGRAPH

The maxillary sinus or antrum is a hollow space within the alveolar bone that contains air. It is one of the sinuses surrounding the nose. Typically, only the bottom half of this cavity is observed on a periapical projection as a radiolucent shadow surrounded by a delicate jagged radiopaque edge. Occasionally, this sinus cavity will expand into the area between the roots of the back teeth and form what looks like a depression. This condition is referred to as pneumatization, and it can be observed with chronic sinus diseases, aging, or early extraction of molars in the maxillary jaw.

READING PANORAMIC RADIOGRAPHS

Individuals who read panoramic radiographs must be familiar with a variety of common anatomical landmarks in the maxillofacial region and other areas of the face in addition to the teeth. These landmarks include bones, arch structures, ridge formations, palates, typical air spaces, and the like.

47

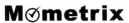

They must also be aware of what types of structures can obscure others on the image and conditions that affect the relative radiolucency of objects. A much larger area is covered on a panoramic radiograph than any other type of dental image. The interplay between the teeth and other structures can be visualized to a large extent, which means pathological conditions can be more easily diagnosed.

RADIOLUCENCIES AND RADIOPACITIES IN PANORAMIC RADIOLOGY

Any object in the path of the x-ray beam can produce single, double, or ghost images depending on its orientation. These objects include not only anatomical or other entities located on the patient, but also parts of the machinery. All of these images are superimposed on the radiograph, but certain types of tissues and materials block out others to an extent. **Radiopaque objects** absorb x-rays and **radiolucent entities** do not in general. Therefore, black air spaces can make it difficult to see hard tissues. Soft and hard tissues are both relatively radiopaque, but hard tissues absorb the radiation to a greater extent and can obscure soft ones. Soft tissues can mask air spaces, and ghost images can be visible over everything else. These concepts can be used to diagnose pathological conditions because changes in an area generally make that region more radiolucent.

LOCALIZING UNERUPTED TEETH AND FOREIGN OBJECTS ON RADIOGRAPH

In general, there are two ways to localize entities like unerupted teeth, foreign bodies, or other irregularities on a radiograph. The first technique is the **tube-shift method of localization** in which a series of periapical radiographs is taken with the tubehead positioned differently horizontally for each. If the object in question shifts in harmony with the tubehead, it is located on the lingual or tongue side. If the entity appears to move in opposition to the tubehead, then it is located on the facial or buccal side. Another principle that can be applied to localization of objects is the **buccal-object rule**. Again, two radiographs of a region are necessary; vertically aligned images are discriminated through changes in horizontal angulation of the x-ray beam while horizontal aligned images are discerned through changes in vertical angulation. Here hidden or unidentified entities that are buccal known objects move in the same direction as the x-ray beam or positioning device, and lingual objects shift in opposition to beam movement.

LANDMARKS ON RADIOGRAPHS THAT HELP DETERMINE BONE HEIGHT

The level of bone on the facial side can be estimated by using the lamina dura. The lamina dura is the portion of the bone seen as a radiopaque line on the radiograph. The point at which it starts to become less opaque or solid is a good approximation of where the interseptal bone begins. The level of bone on the lingual or tongue side is usually determined by finding the faint line that undulates across the center of the teeth. This line distinguishes between the areas of the root that are covered by bone and those that are not and represents the level of the alveolar crest. From the alveolar crest to the apex is the bone height for the lingual aspect.

FURCATION INVOLVEMENT

Teeth further back in the jaw can be bifurcated or trifurcated. In other words, they can have roots that branch or divide into two parts or three parts because the periodontal pocket has enlarged. If there is a pocket in the gum tissue around the root, there is furcation involvement. A radiograph that shows widening of the periodontal ligament space or significant bone loss suggests furcation. Usually, the dentist investigates this condition by inserting a probe into the top of the area (possibly in conjunction with warm condensed air). Furcation involvement can be found near many teeth, but it is observed most often initially in the first molar area.

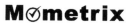

Purpose and Technique

INDICATIONS FOR FURTHER UNCONVENTIONAL RADIOGRAPHIC METHODS

There are four methods of defining the relationship between different structures in the oral cavity. In the first method, two objects are localized by definition on a normal radiograph. In other words, the more defined object is considered to be located lingually on the tongue side because that is the position of the sensor. The tube shift approach compares two radiographs whose only difference is a slight shift of the x-ray tube's horizontal angulation. Here a principle called the buccal-object rule is employed; according to this rule, buccal objects appear to move in the opposite direction. These techniques are also employed to localize foreign objects or unerupted teeth. A similar type of relationship can be found when observing some older pantomographic exposures. Periapical images used in conjunction with occlusal images taken at right angles can provide information about structural relationships as well.

APPEARANCE OF DENTAL DEVICES ON RADIOGRAPHS

ENDODONTIC OR OTHER RESTORATIVE MATERIALS

Various types of foreign restorative materials are inserted into the dental cavity for treatment of endodontic or pulp diseases. These materials can contain silver, gold, a pliable latex substance called gutta percha, or various amalgams (typically mercury, silver, and tin). During the actual endodontic process, other objects like clamps or files might be inserted into the region as well. On a radiograph, all of these materials are observed as intensely radiopaque, even relative to the tooth enamel. Other restorative materials that appear radiopaque can include newer tooth-colored composites and various types of cements. On the other hand, many modern restorations utilize acrylic or composites made with it, and the acrylic is radiolucent. Older porcelain crowns also appear relatively dark on the image, as they lack the strong filler materials that are found in crowns manufactured today.

ORTHODONTIC DEVICES, PEDIATRIC RESTORATIONS, OR PROSTHODONTIC MATERIALS

Most orthodontic devices are bands, wires, brackets, spacers, or retainers containing stainless steel, so they are seen as intensely radiopaque areas on radiographs. Unfortunately, some of these devices obscure evidence of underlying tooth decay. There are also newer clear plastic aligners available, but these would normally be removed before an image is exposed.

Prosthodontic materials like dentures or bridges should also be taken out before radiographs are taken. Again, these devices mask other disease processes if left in; the metallic portions would appear extremely white and the porcelain or acrylic sections would prevent absorption of the radiation and seem darker. Infrequently, materials inserted for hygienic or periodontal purposes may also show up as radiopaque areas on an image.

FOREIGN MATERIALS INSERTED DURING ORAL SURGERY

There are a variety of wires, bars, crowns, bridges, and screws that might be permanently or temporarily inserted into the jaw area during oral surgery. Usually, these insertions are done after some sort of traumatic incident like an automobile accident or explosion. Most of the foreign materials utilized contain a metal, either stainless steel or some type of amalgam, which means that they appear as very white, radiopaque areas on the radiograph. Bone should surround the implant. White fragments visualized on an image can also be clues to a patient's history, because these pieces can remain imbedded.

OTHER TYPES OF FOREIGN MATERIALS SEEN ON RADIOGRAPH

Sometimes devices used during the exposure of a radiograph might appear on the image. For example, RINN XCP devices are often seen as either white regions (if metallic) or relatively dark areas (if plastic). External jewelry, eyeglasses or other materials are generally observed as white

49

areas. In addition, occasionally radiopaque materials are injected into various passages to visualize structures or make them denser; these areas will be light on the radiograph as well.

PERIODONTAL DISEASE

Periodontal disease is a blanket term for processes that change the gums or tissues that envelop and support the teeth. The majority of these diseases are caused by microbial infections resulting from plaque buildup, other pathogenic exposure, restorative work, or tartar. The disease is distinguished by inflamed gums, development of pockets in the area, and damage to the associated ligaments and alveolar bone. Progression of bone loss is diagnostic for periodontitis. Periodontal pockets are grooves of soft tissue that can be identified only by use of probing instruments. If left untreated, periodontal disease can result in tooth loss.

STAGING AND GRADING

Periodontal disease is diagnosed by a combination of methods. The staging phase, as outlined by 2018 AAP guidelines, involves measuring interdental calculus, radiographic bone loss, tooth loss, probing the gums, and assessing bone loss and furcation involvement. Assessing these elements involves a variety of techniques:

- Pockets are generally identified by **probing** with an instrument or by **inserting radiopaque substances** in the area and capturing an image.
- Visualization of bone requires sequential radiography and digital subtraction techniques (a popular feature of digital imaging where the white and black areas can be reversed to indicate pathology otherwise unnoticed.
- Radiographs alone cannot determine the characteristics of the bone deformity. There is also an instrument called the **Nabors probe** that can be used to detect furcation or separation of the tooth from the underlying bone; sometimes this can be seen radiographically as a dark area.
- **Dental calculus or mineralization** can sometimes be picked up as white lines or spurs on exposures.
- **Progression toward tooth loosening** can be diagnosed if the periodontal ligament space gets wider, but this is rarely observable on a radiograph because other structures obscure the changes.

SEQUENTIAL RADIOGRAPHS

Radiographs cannot show depth, and thus bones and teeth are generally visually laid over each other in the image. This means that a single radiograph might pick up bone loss and indicate periodontal disease, but it is not useful in determining the extent or rate of progression of the condition. Small amounts of bone loss are difficult to see on an individual image. On the other hand, if **sequential radiographs** at different time intervals are taken, changes can be visualized using computerized digital subtraction. The two images are digitally merged, the common areas are subtracted out, and the resultant picture shows only the differences. Tiny changes can be measured by this technique. The paralleling method with high voltage and a long positioning device should be used.

INITIAL CHANGES ASSOCIATED WITH PERIODONTAL DISEASE

An early radiographic indication of periodontal disease is the blurring or discontinuity of the lamina dura or bone surrounding the periodontal ligament. These are known as irregularities of the alveolar bone crest. Another early indication is the widening of the periodontal ligament space which can sometimes be seen as a darker triangular or funnel-like area. Radiographs can sometimes pick up early interseptal bone changes as dark protrusions into the alveolar bone

Purpose and Technique

region. The mechanism involved is the expansion of blood vessels in the bone as a result of increased inflammation of the gum. The concentration of minerals in the tissues is decreased as well. Eventually, the teeth may appear to be completely detached from the underlying bone. Calculus deposits may be seen between the surfaces of the teeth.

COMMON FUNCTIONAL PROBLEMS CONTRIBUTING TO PERIODONTAL DISEASE

The two most common functional issues that contribute to periodontal disease development are occlusal traumatism and a high crown-to-root ratio. The occlusal surfaces of the teeth can become traumatized primarily through undesirable oral practices such as grinding of the teeth (known as bruxism) or firmly holding and clenching the teeth. These practices tend to collapse the underlying ligaments, cause bone to reabsorb, enlarge the periodontal ligament space, and eventually lead to loosening of the teeth. Radiographs can aid with clinical diagnosis of occlusal traumatism. In addition, when individuals have teeth with long crowns relative to the root, or a high crown-to-root ratio, the load applied to the gum is high. This condition can be clearly seen on a radiograph, and it is prevalent in the Latin American population.

RISK FACTORS FOR PERIODONTAL DISEASE

Periodontal disease is primarily an inflammatory disease of the gum area caused by buildup of bacterial plaque. There are a number of factors that can predispose an individual toward development of this buildup. A radiograph can only detect these factors; it cannot determine the exact role they may play in development of periodontal disease. The first element is deposition of calculus or tartar, which is the concretion of bacteria and other organic materials on the surface of the tooth. Calculus is often described in terms of where it is found and the source of the other organic materials. Supragingival and subgingival calculus have contributions from saliva and serum respectively. Restorations or implants that are done incorrectly are other significant causes of periodontal disease (now categorized as peri-implant disease) because they can leave overhangs or gaps where bacteria can grow and attach. Similarly, areas that allow food to become impacted or stuck can predispose a person to periodontal disease. Examples of these types of areas include sections that have worn away on the tooth surface or are decayed.

USE OF RADIOGRAPHS TO DETERMINE RATE OF PERIODONTAL DAMAGE

Periodontal damage can be an active or relatively static process, and radiographs are useful for determination of the **rate of destruction of the gum area**. The appearance of the crests of the interseptal alveolar bone is generally used to assess the activity level. If this crest is uneven and less defined, the periodontal destruction is probably active. If on the other hand, the crest is smooth, distinct, and relatively radiopaque, the gingival breakdown is not active at that time. Usually, diagnosis is made by comparing sequential radiographs. The prognosis or final outcome can only be estimated by assimilation of all available data, which should include radiographs and clinical evaluation.

BONE LOSS
DETERMINING BONE LOSS WITH RADIOGRAPHS

Bone loss is actually evaluated by comparing the amount of enduring bone to the expected amount of bone. The most common site for initial evaluation is the interproximal septal bone. The cementoenamel junction (CEJ) is the part of the tooth where the enamel ends and the dentin starts. The distance from that point towards the apex of the tooth is normally 1.0-1.5 millimeters; therefore, bone loss is measured as the difference between the observed height and the expected height. Bone loss can be generalized (evident consistently on the majority of teeth), or it can be localized to only certain teeth. In either case, inflammatory processes resulting from periodontitis

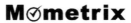

usually occur concurrently, and thus loss of contact between the dentition is also observed on the radiograph.

DIRECTION OF BONE LOSS

Bone loss can occur in different planes. If the deficiency is generally found in the plane equidistant from the CEJ of adjoining teeth, the loss is considered horizontal. If the **pattern of bone loss** is more angular and inconsistent between adjacent teeth, the loss is defined as vertical or angular. The latter configuration may also show enlargement of the periodontal ligament space or pockets below the bone. Both types of bone loss probably involve local inflammatory responses, but a vertical pattern may indicate systemic involvement as well. Evidence of vertical bone loss without accompanying plaque buildup or gingivitis in teenagers is called localized juvenile periodontitis (LJP). LJP often occurs in the premolar-molar region and the rate of bone loss can be very high. The etiology of LJP is unclear, but it is probably infectious or immunologic in nature.

INFRABONY POCKETS

Infrabony pockets are regions created through crestal bone loss and observed on radiographs as dark areas protruding into the bone area between the teeth. These pockets or defects extend below the level of the adjacent alveolar crest and typically have one, two, or three bone walls. A one-wall or hemiseptum defect occurs when only one wall of the interseptal bone is damaged leaving the other intact. Two-wall infrabony pockets are the most common type, in particular a variant called an osseous crater, which constitutes over half of all defects in the lower jaw. An osseous crater appears on the radiograph as a concave indentation in the bone between two teeth. A three-wall pocket is bounded by three bony walls and the root, and a four-wall defect entirely encompasses the root area. Usually, these defects are confirmed by probing with an instrument.

DENTAL CARIES

Dental caries or tooth decay is the breakdown of hard dentin tissue in a tooth. Caries development is dependent on three aspects. All must be present for tooth decay to occur.

- First, the host must have a propensity towards caries development.
- Then, specific bacteria or microflora must be present.
- Lastly, dietary sugars that can ferment or be broken down into acids and other substances must be available. The acids are the substances that actually demineralize or decalcify and break down the hard enamel of the tooth. As the breakdown proceeds over time, eventually tooth decay or caries can be detected.

Typically, radiographic visualization occurs when about half the calcium and phosphorus is broken down.

INTERPROXIMAL ENAMEL CARIES

Interproximal enamel caries is the tooth decay that occurs between two abutting tooth surfaces. Initially, interproximal enamel caries starts just underneath the point of contact. At this point, the lesion looks white and chalky, and a small dark notch is visible on a radiograph. As the destruction proceeds, the shape of the lesion usually becomes an elongated triangle. The longer tip of the triangle is directed downward toward the dentinoenamel junction (DEJ). Caries visualization on a radiograph is influenced by the spatial parameters of the adjoining tooth, in particular the area of the contact point which can obscure the extent of the decay.

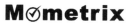

TYPES

There are several types of interproximal enamel caries that do not have the characteristic triangular appearance running along the edge of the tooth.

- One is **incipient caries**, which is decay that has not completely penetrated the enamel. On a radiograph, incipient caries usually looks like a small, dark funnel-shaped area.
- Another type is **lamellar caries**, which appears as a dark line that progresses into the dentin region.
- There can also be decay primarily within the dentin called **dentinal caries**. This type of decay looks restricted to areas under the enamel on a radiograph, and it can destroy tubules in the dentin.

ACUTE VS. CHRONIC CARIES

The terms acute and chronic as applied to dental caries differentiate between the rates of penetration of the lesion, in other words fast versus slow. In addition, acute caries tends to arise from a relatively tiny surface point compared to chronic cases. Tooth decay in younger people tends to proceed more rapidly than in older individuals. For example, a condition called rampant caries, in which the decay has an abrupt onset and extremely rapid progression, commonly occurs only in children and adolescents. Rampant caries is rarely found in adults, except in some cases of xerostomia or dry mouth. Acute caries is prevalent from adolescence to about age 25, and chronic tooth decay is usually the type found above that age range.

RADIOGRAPHIC CLASSIFICATION SYSTEM FOR DENTAL CARIES

The extent of dental caries is currently classified into 4 groups depending on the penetration of the destruction as visualized on a radiograph. The decision to treat caries should be based upon the combination of this radiographic classification and clinical evaluation.

- **Incipient**: Enamel is penetrated by a lesion less than halfway.
- **Moderate**: Enamel is penetrated by a lesion more than halfway.
- **Advanced**: Enamel is fully penetrated at least to the DEJ, but not more than halfway to the pulp.
- **Severe**: Lesion extends through enamel, dentin, and more than halfway to the pulp.

RADIOGRAPHIC APPEARANCE OF CARIES ON FACIAL OR LINGUAL SIDES OF TOOTH

Tooth decay can occur on the facial or lingual sides of the tooth as well as the neck or cervical region of the crown. The point of entrance of the caries is usually relatively large compared to other decay types. These types of lesions are visualized as very well-defined radiolucent circular areas on the radiograph generally, although they might also appear as dark oval or arc shapes. Caries on these surfaces is hard to detect until it has progressed to a certain point. These smooth surface types of caries are usually identified by using a mirror and some type of exploratory probe.

OCCLUSAL CARIES

Caries that begins on the occlusal surface of a tooth is extremely common in younger patients, particularly in the molar and pre-molar regions. The occlusal surfaces of teeth in these areas are very uneven and layered deeply with enamel. Poor dental hygiene in the back of the mouth and lack of preventive measures including dental sealants increase the possibility of caries in this area. Occlusal tooth decay is usually not detected on a radiograph until it has broken through the dentinoenamel junction (DEJ), at which point it appears as a dark line or region just below the DEJ. Actually, the caries spreads up into the enamel as well. Therefore, mirrors and certain probes are usually used to identify cases of occlusal caries.

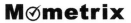

ROOT CARIES

Tooth decay can occur in the root area of the tooth without enamel involvement. This type of root or cemental caries usually begins in the cementoenamel junction or CEJ region as a result of plaque retention along receding gums. The caries usually radiates outward from the point of origin, eventually merging into a circular area. Radiographically the decay appears to engulf and blur the entire root area, and clinically it erodes the cementum located at the CEJ. The enamel is not directly affected, but cemental caries can broaden into regions very close to it. Root caries is prevalent in the elderly population.

PULPAL CARIES

A radiograph is of limited value in the diagnostic evaluation of pulpal caries. Pulpal caries is decay that has extended into the central tooth pulp, which contains nerve endings and blood vessels. Since radiographs cannot show depth, it is very difficult to angle the beam to pick up pulp involvement without creating other distortions. In particular, the exposure may obscure the extent or absence of pulpal involvement because the radiolucent decay area is shown over the pulp. This distortion is exaggerated further if the picture is overexposed.

RADIATION CARIES

Radiation caries is the progressive decay of teeth or bones in the maxillofacial region after high dose radiation treatment of head or neck cancer. When doses of about 6000 rad are used to kill cancerous cells in the region, the softer tissues like the salivary glands are often affected as well. The amount of saliva produced is depleted and it becomes thicker decreasing the ability of saliva to clean the teeth and keep the mouth moist. Friction in the mouth and the predilection towards development of caries are both increased. Another condition called osteoradionecrosis, or destruction of bone tissue, may also develop.

HALTED CARIES

Various types of caries can be halted or arrested if the environmental milieu changes into one that does not promote decay. Incipient caries, in which the decay has not penetrated much of the enamel, is common, and typically the enamel is as hard as that in a healthy tooth. The mechanism in this case is probably remineralization of the enamel. This type of arrested caries is often seen adjacent to another tooth that has been removed. Sometimes tooth decay on occlusal surfaces stops because the dentin has become so hard upon repeated buffing that bacteria are sloughed off. In this case, there is a characteristic radiographic appearance including a missing crown with a ragged, radiolucent space in its place.

SECONDARY CARIES

Secondary caries is tooth decay that emerges after restorations of previous caries have been in place for a period of time. It is usually visualized on a radiograph as a dark radiolucent spot near the restoration. The secondary or recurrent caries can have two different types of causes. In some cases, dentitional caries in the hard part of the tooth under the enamel was not entirely eradicated before the restoration was done. New caries can also develop if tin or zinc leaks out from the filling or cement. In the latter case, the current theory is that the metal ions combine with demineralized dentin to initiate fresh areas of decay.

CERVICAL BURNOUT

Cervical burnout is an artifact that appears to be caries on an exposure. The cervical neck of the tooth is tapered. Therefore, it attracts fewer energy photons and appears darker on a radiograph than the crown above or root below it. Thus, a radiolucent band or collar may be observed on a radiograph, but there is actually no decay. In the posterior teeth, the radiographic appearance of

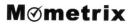

cervical burnout can be more pie-shaped. Similar contrast artifacts may be observed at the cementoenamel junction, with certain root arrangements, or if the beam is directed incorrectly horizontally. Correct horizontal angulation usually eliminates cervical burnout.

REASONS THAT THE EXTENT OF CARIES CAN BE OVERLOOKED

The relative thickness of the tooth and its area of decay can influence interpretation of the extent of caries on a radiograph. X-ray beams are impeded and absorbed by interaction with the enamel. In areas where the carious lesion is narrowing, such as where it may be entering the dentin, the large enamel area can obscure the much smaller radiolucent decay area. In addition, at least half the calcium and phosphorus must be destroyed before a lesion can be visualized on a radiograph, a trait that leads to inherent underestimation of caries involvement.

CONDITIONS OF THE TOOTH ENAMEL THAT LOOK LIKE CARIES ON A RADIOGRAPH

Areas of the tooth can be mechanically worn down and look like caries on a radiograph. One type of corrosion is called attrition, in which occlusal or incisal edges are worn down. If the attrition is severe enough to include dentin involvement, a hollow space that appears to be caries can develop. The other type of corrosion that mimics decay is called abrasion, and it is usually observed in the root area with receding gums. In addition, there is a condition called enamel hypoplasia in which incomplete development results in fissures in the enamel. These fissures may stain and appear to be decay. Enamel hypoplasia can be distinguished from caries by using an exploratory probe; the probe detaches easily in hypoplasia but does not with true caries.

RESTORATIVE DENTAL MATERIALS THAT MAY RESEMBLE CARIES

Restorative dental materials made from substances that are also radiolucent like decay can resemble caries formation on a radiograph. In general, this situation only occurs when the restoration is relatively old and materials like certain plastics, silicates, or calcium hydroxide were used. The cements used to affix these materials generally contain metals, however; the adjacent cement appears as a white area on the exposure and aids in differentiation between these materials and true decay. Newer restorations generally are comprised of high molecular weight metals, either gold or amalgam mixtures, rendering them radiopaque. Thus, newer dental work is rarely confused with caries.

PULPITIS

The pulp chamber and its canal are areas in the middle of the crown and root of the tooth. Generally, they do not contain calcified materials like bones do, and therefore they appear as radiolucent areas on a radiograph. The configuration of the pulp area is reduced with aging, in a few developmental abnormalities, or if the area is irritated. Dentin is deposited on the walls of the area as well during these processes. If there is irritation from decay or other trauma, the result is a condition called pulpitis. Pulpitis cannot generally be identified on a radiograph. Occasionally, there may be small areas with calcification in the pulp chamber that show up as radiopaque regions, but in general they have no clinical significance.

PERIAPICAL DISEASE

Periapical disease is any disruption of the lamina dura at the apex of a tooth. The lamina dura is the cortical bone surrounding the periodontal ligament. Healthy individuals have dense lamina dura that appears radiographically as a narrow, white line running near the apex of the tooth. When the line loses its continuous appearance due to resorption of the lamina dura and alveolar bone, some sort of periapical disease exists. The classification of the type of periapical disease generally requires additional clinical investigation. Some periapical diseases are acutely symptomatic with

55

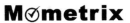

pain and edema, but others persist chronically without significant clinical signs. Many of these conditions are actually periodontal disease as well.

ACUTE APICAL PERIODONTITIS

Acute apical (or periapical) periodontitis, also known as AAP, is inflammation in the region of the periodontal ligament near the apex of the tooth. Clinically, the area is extremely painful, especially if tapped. Often, there is no change seen on a radiograph in the lamina dura or periodontal ligament spaces, although the latter may be wider than usual. There can be a variety of reasons for this inflammation. The most common causes are either some sort of irritation derived from pulpitis traveling via the root canal or response to some injury or foreign material (including restorations). If pulpitis is the causative agent, the damage is irreparable, the pulp tissue may be dead, and the pulp may need to be removed and a root canal procedure performed.

ACUTE APICAL ABSCESS

If acute apical periodontitis caused by a dead tooth pulp is left untreated, an acute apical abscess (AAA) can develop. The infection is evidenced by pus accumulated at the apex of the root, generalized pain and edema in the area, and pain and tenderness on percussion. Eventually, the tooth can come out of its socket and move around. The purulent exudate must be drained immediately to alleviate symptoms. On a radiograph, an early AAA may be difficult to pinpoint. Changes to look for include an expansion of the periodontal ligament space. Advanced cases can show dark areas where the alveolar bone has been damaged.

CHRONIC APICAL ABSCESS

A chronic apical abscess (CAA) is the end-result of a persistent acute apical abscess. It is often identified because a tooth is loose, or gum tissues are tender or swollen. As with the AAA, the pulp is dead, and an infection is present in the apical area. A glaucomatous sac surrounds the purulent materials. There are two ways that chronic apical abscesses present themselves, and they are differentiated by the route for pus drainage. Most CAAs form canals or fistulas from the abscessed area through the alveolar bone to the outside of the gum where a boil or parulis is formed. Drainage of the CAA is generally then performed through this boil to alleviate the swelling and pain. On a radiograph, the fistula looks like a dark channel. Sometimes the chronic apical abscess does not form a fistula and the purulent material drains internally into the circulatory or lymphatic systems. For this type of CAA, the radiolucent sac has very indistinct borders indicating dispersion into other areas. In either type of CAA, a root canal procedure is indicated.

APICAL GRANULOMA

When apical periodontitis becomes chronic, an apical granuloma may form as a mechanism to confine the irritants from the dead pulp and root canal. Essentially, a fibrous pouch forms along the periodontal ligament around the chronically inflamed tissue in the apical area. Clinically, this sac formation relieves some of the pain and may arrest pustule formation, but generally root canal procedures are still necessary to prevent tooth loss. On a radiograph, an apical granuloma looks like a small dark rounded or oval area protruding from the apical area of the tooth. In the molar area of the upper jaw, this condition may cause the mucosal membranes of the sinus to become inflamed as well; this is known as antral mucositis.

APICAL CYST

When an apical granuloma expands in size, an apical cyst can form within the granuloma. The apical cyst consists of layers of squamous or scale-shaped epithelial cells that form a sac filled with liquid. Pressure builds up within the cyst, and bone near the apex is resorbed. Clinically, the area may not hurt unless it has become infected. Nevertheless, all irritating substances in the dead pulp are

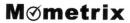

generally eradicated, and the root canal is closed up. Cysts are relatively easy to recognize on a radiograph because they appear as large radiolucent areas attached to the apex of the tooth and rimmed by a radiopaque outline of the bone.

APICAL CONDENSING OSTEITIS

Apical condensing osteitis (ACO) is dense bone formation in the apical tooth area that occurs in response to low-grade bacterial infection of the pulp. The alveolar bone is not actually destroyed in ACO. The condition is often asymptomatic but probing, and other types of stimuli indicate that the pulp tissue is necrosed. On a radiograph, radiopaque areas are observed near the tooth apex. Condensing osteitis is prevalent in the premolar and molar regions of the mandible. As with other apical conditions, root canal treatment is generally performed in these patients.

BENIGN CONDITIONS IN THE APICAL REGION

Apical cementoma, also called periapical cementoma or cemental dysphasia, is a disorder in which connective tissues overgrow and destroy the lamina dura. The lesions themselves emanate from the periapical area and appear dark on a radiograph with possible radiopaque infill containing cementum or bone during more advanced stages. Since pulp is not destroyed in this condition, the teeth are alive, and no root canal or other type of management is necessary. Another benign condition of the apical area is hypercementosis, in which excessive amounts of cementum deposit along the root of the tooth. On a radiograph, hypercementosis presents as either generalized enlargement of the root area or a nodule on the tip of the root.

ABNORMAL DENTITION NUMBERS

There are a number of developmental aberrations in which the normal distribution or appearance of teeth is not seen. If the normal number of teeth is not observed, there are three possible conditions.

- **Anodontia** is a genetic disorder in which no teeth ever develop. People with anodontia are said to be edentulous.
- **Hypodontia** is a genetic condition in which one or more teeth are missing. If many teeth are missing, the condition is sometimes referred to as oligodontia.
- **Hyperdontia** is a genetic condition in which additional teeth are present. The extra teeth are also termed supernumerary.

DIVISION OR FUSION ERRORS RESULTING IN ABNORMAL DENTITION NUMBER

There are several conditions where division or fusion errors give the appearance of an abnormal dentition number. Two of these alterations are primarily observed in the front incisors.

- **Gemination** occurs when an individual tooth bud tries to split, but the division only occurs near the top. This gives the appearance of two teeth near the crown, but there is a common root canal.
- When two adjoining teeth join at the dentin and/or enamel areas, a process called **fusion** occurs. This condition reduces the total number of teeth observed, but a radiograph shows that there are actually two separate root canals.

ABNORMAL TEETH SIZE

Teeth can be larger or smaller than expected.

- Relatively large dentition, termed **macrodontia**, is not very common. Pituitary giants experience generalized macrodontia, but other people may have individual teeth that are enlarged. Individuals with diminutive jaws appear to have macrodontia.
- Some people have **microdontia** in which all or some of the teeth are abnormally small relative to jaw size. The most common examples are small lateral incisors in the maxilla, a condition that tends to segregate in families, or small third molars. Microdontia is seen in pituitary dwarfs.

TAURODONTISM AND SUPERNUMERARY ROOTS

Both taurodontism and supernumerary roots are conditions in which the shape of root area of the tooth has developed abnormally. In **taurodontism**, the root is abbreviated and the pulp compartment is enlarged, giving a squared-off appearance to the apical area. **Supernumerary roots** are additional roots on a tooth giving a branching appearance on a radiograph. Sometimes there are separate relatively small root canals in each branch as well. The number of branches is typically two or three. The periodontal ligament spaces can shift with supernumerary roots. This condition is most common in the canine and pre-molar regions of the lower jaw.

IMPACT OF TOOTH SHAPE CHANGES ON EXTRACTION AND ORTHODONTIC PROBLEMS

Adjacent teeth can join in the cementum region during root growth or eruption (occasionally later), and this phenomenon is known as **concrescence**. The most common sites for concrescence are various molars, particularly in the maxilla. The lack of separation and distorted relationship makes tooth extraction and corrective procedures very problematic in these teeth. Teeth can also be bent, particularly in the root area but sometimes in the crown. These curved shape changes are called dilacerations, and they can have a myriad of causes that are usually traumatic in nature. If a tooth is bent, the teeth in the area can be positioned incorrectly which again interferes with orthodontia or extraction.

DENS INVAGINATUS AND DENS EVAGINATUS

Dens invaginatus and dens evaginatus are both abnormalities in the pattern of the folding of the enamel at the occlusal surface. In dens invaginatus (also called dens in dente), the enamel on the crown folds inward, leaving a hollow. This anomaly is relatively common. Since this invagination makes the pulp more vulnerable to exposure and the tooth more prone to decay, the crater is often closed up during youth. In dens evaginatus (also known as Leong's premolar), the enamel on the crown folds outward, creating a bump. During dental probing, teeth with this type of elevation can be subjected to mechanical and inflammatory stresses, so decay and pulp problems can occur here as well.

ENAMEL PEARLS

Enamel pearls are tiny spherical or oval pieces of enamel that adhere to the outside of the tooth. They are usually found in the molar region on the cervical neck of the tooth or in areas where branching has occurred. Since these pearls or enamelomas are made of enamel, they appear as opaque dots on a radiograph when observed in certain orientations that do not obscure them. Enamel pearls originating at branching points predispose an individual to periodontal disease if they are not removed because a pocket can form at the furcation. Enamel pearls can be confused radiographically with calcified areas in the pulp because both are radiopaque. The two can be distinguished by the fact that pulpal calcifications will be seen in various orientations whereas enamelomas will not.

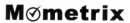

AMELOGENESIS IMPERFECTA

If defective enamel formation or enamel hypoplasia is **inherited**, it is called amelogenesis imperfecta. Tooth decay is rare in individuals with this hereditary alteration. There are three types of amelogenesis imperfecta.

- In the first **hypoplastic variation**, the enamel's structure is unaltered, but the width of its layer is very narrow.
- In the **hypomineralized deviation**, the concentration of minerals in the enamel is low, which renders the tooth susceptible to pitting or splintering.
- The third variant is the **hypomaturation type** in which the grinding surface of the tooth has a white or pitted tip.

DENTINOGENESIS IMPERFECTA

Dentinogenesis imperfecta is an inherited abnormality that involves the dentin and its connection with the enamel. The teeth have a shimmery appearance and they tend to crack. There are three classifications of dentinogenesis imperfecta differentiated primarily in terms of the association or lack thereof between generalized bone disease and changes in the tooth structure.

- **Type 1** occurs in individuals who also have generalized bone disease or osteogenesis imperfecta. In the other manifestations, this disorder only affects the teeth.
- **Type 2** can be seen in the general population without other inherited disorders.
- The more severe **Type 3** occurs only in restricted populations in the eastern United States. On a radiograph, the pulp area looks destroyed, and the roots are shortened and narrow with no evidence of a root canal.

ENAMEL HYPOPLASIA

Any condition in which the milieu of the enamel has been altered is called enamel hypoplasia. There are a number of possible manifestations of flawed enamel formation. If the alteration is localized to a single tooth as a pitted appearance, the causative agent was probably external trauma or infection. In baby teeth, this anomaly is often referred to as Turner's tooth. If a child is malnourished or contracts certain infections that produce a high fever, they can develop pitting or enamel hypoplasia on all or the majority of their teeth. This condition can develop in both primary incisors as well as permanent incisors if the deficiency or infection occurs during the first two years of life. Excessive exposure to fluorine can also produce another form of enamel hyperplasia in which the tooth surface appears mottled or discolored.

DENTAL DYSPLASIAS

A dysplasia is some type of unusual growth or absence of a part. Two types of dysplasias are found in dentition.

- One is **dentinal dysplasia** in which the enamel appears normal but underneath the pulp and root areas are either defective or destroyed. Root development is minimal with this abnormality.
- In another type of dysphasia called **regional odontodysplasia**, both the dentin and enamel do not develop properly, and the delineation between them disappears. Thus, on a radiograph, the tooth is less radiopaque and has a ghost-like appearance. The pulp cavity also looks relatively large.

Both of these conditions are uncommon.

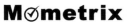

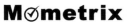

ABNORMALITIES DURING TOOTH ERUPTION

Tooth eruption is the time period when the tooth emerges through the gum. If the tooth migrates or moves in a strange pattern prior to eruption, it will remain buried within the jawbone. If the tooth moves after it has erupted, contact between normally adjacent teeth may be lost and this is referred to as **drift**. Teeth can also exchange normal positions upon eruption, a condition known as **translocation**. Translocation is usually not a major issue because no crowding or dental arch changes occur. On the other hand, sometimes a tooth can break out into an abnormal position. This situation, known as **ectopic eruption**, can create space problems and change the shape of the arch. Another condition, especially prevalent in the third molar region, is **tooth impaction**. Here, some spatial impedance such as another tooth changes the orientation of the imbedded tooth making eruption impossible; these teeth are usually extracted.

ACQUIRED TOOTH DEFECTS

Tooth defects can be initiated through various types of **mechanical or chemical wear and tear**.

- **Attrition** and **abrasion** can look like tooth decay on a radiograph. Attrition is the wearing away of teeth by normal occlusal forces, whereas abrasion is wearing away by a mechanical device that has been introduced into the area. These mechanical devices include things like workplace items (for example, a hairdresser puts hairpins in her mouth), toothbrushes used incorrectly, ritual insertions into the oral cavity, and cocaine use. The abrasive pattern depends on the item used, but in all cases a radiolucent area is observed on a radiograph.
- **Erosion** or the chemical breakdown of the tooth's surface can also occur, possibly revealing the dentin underneath. Many of the causes involve exposure to acids from medications or soda. Disorders of the digestive tract like bulimia or vomiting often lead to tooth erosion. On a radiograph, the crowns may look darker if erosion has occurred.

CLEFT PALATE

A cleft is a narrow surface indentation that occurs because certain embryonic processes failed to fuse during development. In the context of dentistry, clefts can be found in the roof of the mouth, in either the bony front hard palate, the soft muscular palate located further back, or possibly in both. On a radiograph, the cleft area is radiolucent. Other developmental abnormalities can be found in conjunction with a cleft palate because the bones are shifted. Malpositioning is common as well as changes in the number of teeth ranging from complete anodontia to extra supernumerary dentition.

FISSURAL AND DENTIGEROUS CYSTS

A cyst is any type of bone cavity lined with epithelial cells. Fissural cysts are sacs that emerge along embryonic junctures. There are three types of typical **fissural cysts**, each with a characteristic position. All look like radiolucent sacs on a radiograph.

- The **nasopalatine cyst** is typically located along the midline adjacent to the apices of incisors in the upper jaw.
- Further back along the midline, a **median palatine cyst** can occur.
- A **globulomaxillary cyst** is more elongated and is found between the lateral incisor and canine in the maxilla.

A **dentigerous cyst** has a completely different origin; it occurs (usually in the third molar) when a tooth bud degenerates to form a cyst or sac. Again, a dark sac is observed on a radiograph.

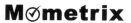

FRACTURES AND EMBEDDED STRUCTURES

Fractures to any part of the tooth appear as dark lines on a radiograph. If they occur in the crown area, they are easily recognizable. Cracks in the root area are more difficult to visualize because the alveolar bone is also in the area. Identification of fractures is important, because pulp damage can lead to other undesirable pathology. Most foreign bodies like implants contain metal and are readily identifiable because they are very radiopaque. Root tips can sometimes be embedded within the jaw and should be removed; they can be found by looking for their canal or their funnel-like shape.

CLASSIFYING UNKNOWN LESIONS

Areas that appear abnormal on a radiograph, but are not easily identified, can be tumors or cysts. A **benign tumor** is not cancerous, does not grow rapidly, and is usually not life-threatening. On a radiograph, a benign tumor presents as a dark, well-defined area. Other structures may be moved around on the radiograph, but they are not destroyed. Conversely, a **malignant tumor** is cancerous and fast-growing, and it does participate in the destruction of other processes. Thus, on a radiograph, a malignant tumor is relatively radiolucent but generally more diffuse and the borders between the malignancy and other structures are less distinct. Tumors can also be radiopaque on the exposure if the density of the tumor tissue is higher than that in the type of cells it is infiltrating, such as bone or cartilage.

SALIVARY STONES

Calcifications, or salivary stones, can occur in the soft tissues of the salivary glands and associated ducts. They can predispose an individual to infection, edema, and obstruction. Thus, even though they do not directly affect the teeth, salivary stones do have diagnostic significance. The stones are easily visualized on radiographs as intensely radiopaque spots. Because of their position, salivary stones are usually identified on occlusal or panoramic images, although they can sometimes be seen on periapical exposures. Salivary stones can also be visualized by injecting radiopaque media into the salivary ducts and glands, a technique called sialography.

UNIVERSAL TOOTH NUMBERING FOR PRIMARY AND PERMANENT TEETH

The universal numbering system is used throughout the United States and is a system that can be recognized across dentistry. This is advantageous especially when patient notes and files are transferred from one dental practice to another or for referrals. All dental offices involved will understand what tooth or teeth are being described in the patients notes.

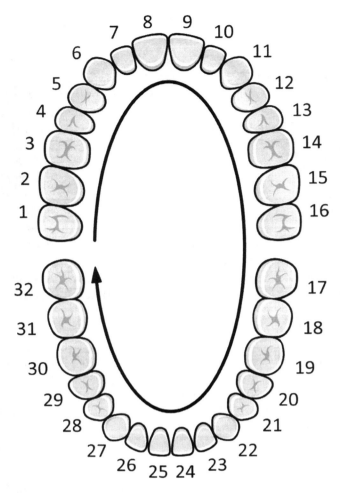

When using the universal numbering system to identify teeth in the adult dentition, each tooth is given a number from 1 through 32. Tooth number 1 is the most upper right molar, moving across the upper arch to tooth number 16, being the farthest upper left molar. Tooth number 17 is identified as the lower left farthest molar, then moving across the lower arch to tooth 32, the tooth that is furthest to the right on the lower arch. The dental team must understand that when referring to teeth using this system, they must include all teeth, even if they are not present in the mouth and must indicate the absent tooth or teeth in the patient's chart. When using this system to identify teeth in the primary dentition, the order of assignment of teeth to a name does not change, but a letter is assigned versus a number. Starting in the upper right with the primary 2nd molar, it is tooth A. The letters then move from the upper right to the upper left, with the left 2nd molar being assigned the name tooth J. Moving down to the lower arch, the lower molar in the far left is tooth K, then moving across to the lower right, the final tooth is T. There are periods of time where an adolescent is in a mixed dentition period, having both priary and permanent teeth present at the same time. The dental team must use both numbers and letters when identifying the teeth present in this mixed dentition.

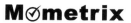

Diagnostically Acceptable Images

DETERMINING DIAGNOSTIC QUALITY OF A DENTAL RADIOGRAPH

The diagnostic or radiographic quality of a dental radiograph is the exactitude of the representation of anatomical structures and their clarity that is visible on the final image. This clarity is comprised of the sharpness or definition of the various structures that are present plus the detail or micro-architecture of these structures. Quality radiographs should demonstrate the proper density and contrast, they should be anatomically correct, they should include all areas of interest, and they need to be sharp. Sharpness or definition can be improved by minimizing distortion and various inherent impediments as well as by controlling magnification.

CRITERIA FOR JUDGING RADIOGRAPHIC IMAGE QUALITY

Radiographic image quality is judged by a number of interrelated characteristics. The radiograph should have enough **detail** to differentiate between various components on the image as well as sufficient **definition** to show structural characteristics and clear demarcation between the components. In general, the latter characteristic, definition, is adequate when surrounding spaces are distinct from the teeth being documented. While detail is primarily controlled by the potential difference applied, and to an extent the development procedures, definition is more a function of factors that can be controlled by the operator such as patient movement, or length of the positioning device. The darkness of the image in general is the density, which should be in a range where surrounding tissues can be faintly observed; it is affected by a number of parameters. A related characteristic is contrast, which is the differentiation in densities between adjoining areas. This factor is primarily determined by the voltage applied. Suitable contrast is important for observation of smaller details and tooth decay. In addition, there should be no significant handling or development errors visible.

CRITERIA FOR JUDGING RADIOGRAPHIC STRUCTURES AND DISTORTION

In a full mouth survey, the tip of every tooth and its adjoining bone should be observed on at least one of the x-rays. For documentation of particular regions, all spaces between, surrounding and/or retromolar to the teeth desired should be visible on the film. Partial images as a result of cone cutting are unacceptable. The cutting edge of the tooth should be oriented toward the raised bump on the film. Distortion of the comparative size and shape of structures should be kept to a minimum. For bitewing radiographs, interproximal connections should be distinct, the visible parts of the teeth in both jaws should be in the center, the peak of the alveolar bone should be visible and differentiated from the teeth, and the biting surface of the teeth should be horizontal. On the other hand, the molar ridges or cusps should be somewhat overlapping.

RESOLUTION OF DIGITAL IMAGES

GRAY-LEVEL RESOLUTION ON DIGITAL IMAGES

Gray-level resolution is the total number of shades of gray that a particular digital image is capable of displaying. Every pixel in the image has an assigned number, which is related to the computer storage capacity. Each bit of computer storage capacity exponentially increases the gray scale resolution according to the formula 2^x where x is number of bits of storage capacity. While current computers may have up to 12 bits or more of storage space, 8 bits are shown on the monitor generally. Since 8 bits represents 2^8 or 256 shades of gray, considerably more than can be distinguished by the human eye, this is sufficient. The numbering is represented as 0 for pure black up to 255 for pure white.

63

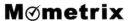

SPATIAL RESOLUTION ON DIGITAL IMAGES

The spatial resolution of a digital image refers to the number of pixels used to create the image. An image with high spatial resolution has more pixels per a specified dimension than an image that has less pixels per the same dimension (low spatial resolution). Resultingly, an image with high spatial resolution is clearer/more detailed than one with low spatial resolution. Spatial resolution as it applies to dental imagery is important in declaring the image's ability to show the required level of detail for abnormalities to be identified and diagnosed.

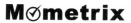

Legal Requirements for Maintaining Dental Images

HIPAA REGULATIONS

The HIPAA or the Health Insurance Portability and Accountability Act of 1996 has three sections: (1) privacy standards, (2) patients' rights, and (3) administrative requirements. The Act requires electronic standardization of patient health care data. The privacy standards section deals primarily with protected health information or PHI. It requires the professional to obtain authorization from the patient before health information can be disclosed for treatment, payment, or healthcare related procedures. This can be in the form of written consent, or they can sign an Acknowledgment of Receipt Notice of Privacy Practices. There are only a few exceptions to these requirements such possible child abuse. Non-adherence can result in civil penalties, fines, or criminal punishments.

ADMINISTRATIVE REQUIREMENTS

The administrative requirements section of the HIPAA mandates that dental offices have a written privacy policy, which can be distributed to the patient. It also requires the dentist to train and familiarize the other personnel in details of the privacy policy and means of documentation. This section also compels the dentist to appoint an office privacy officer to monitor these policies, and another individual to handle complaints. A Notice of Privacy Practices must be in place. If third parties are to have access to patient information, they must be clearly acknowledged as well.

PATIENTS' RIGHTS

The patients' rights section of the HIPAA deals with the entitlements of patients or their representative to obtain their health information. The essence of patients' rights is that they can look at their records, copy them, question violations of rules, and request non-electronic forms of transmission. For minors, these rights generally apply to their parents unless there has been another legal edict. In addition, if the healthcare or dental professional wants to release any information for reason besides treatment, payment, or operations, they must inform the patient.

PREPARING IMAGES FOR LEGAL REQUIREMENTS, DUPLICATION, AND TRANSFER

Dental images may be transferred to other dental practitioners upon written request by the patient, but the original images and dental records remain the property of the originating dentist, who should retain them indefinitely. Patients may ask for copies of records and radiographs but may need to pay a reasonable fee determined by the dental office, especially if an entire record is involved. The patient should not be required to undergo additional imaging to produce new originals. Duplicated images should be mounted and labeled as appropriate. The images and dental records should generally be transferred directly to other dental practitioners through carrier, mail, or internet and not given to the patient to carry, although patients do have that right if they insist. With the use of digital imaging, dental offices can now send patient radiographs through secure electronic files, preventing the need to copy images or use carrier mail.

LEGAL IMPLICATIONS OF BILLING AND PATIENT'S RIGHTS TO OBTAIN X-RAYS

There is legal precedence of the opinion that radiographs are owned by the dental facility generating them, not the patient. By themselves, radiographs are of little value to the patient who is not adept at interpreting them. Therefore, **billing for radiographs** should always be bundled with the cost of dental diagnosis and treatment to avoid the issue of ownership. Negligence claims or malpractice suits can occur if radiographs are delivered to the patient or if they are not applied diagnostically. A radiograph can be submitted as factual evidence in certain legal situations and should therefore always be high-quality. On the other hand, while a dentist is not legally compelled to send completed radiographs to other dentists upon request, they may transmit duplicates via certified or registered mail upon written solicitation by the second practice.

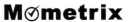

Chapter Quiz

Ready to see how well you retained what you just read? Scan the QR code to go directly to the chapter quiz interface for this study guide. If you're using a computer, simply visit the bonus page at **mometrix.com/bonus948/danbrhs** and click the Chapter Quizzes link.

Radiation Protection

Transform passive reading into active learning! After immersing yourself in this chapter, put your comprehension to the test by taking a quiz. The insights you gained will stay with you longer this way. Scan the QR code to go directly to the chapter quiz interface for this study guide. If you're using a computer, simply visit the bonus page at **mometrix.com/bonus948/danbrhs** and click the Chapter Quizzes link.

Factors Affecting X-Radiation Production and Characteristics

LATENT IMAGE

In direct digital imaging, there is a brief pause from when the exposure button is activated to when the digital image appears on the computer monitor. This can be referred to as a latent image, which is the image that is formed by the radiation, the sensor, and the structures but not is yet visible. When capturing images using indirect digital imaging techniques, the dental assistant must expose the image and then process that image in a digital processor before it is visible on the computer screen. This time from when the image is captured to the time it appears is the latent image.

BENSON LINE FOCUS PRINCIPLE

The path of x-rays can be deflected, and this property is exploited in the design of dental x-ray tubes to sharpen images. The Benson line focus principle reduces the effective dimensions of the focal spot. This is accomplished by an anode design with an angled face to the electron path, typically at 15-20° relative to the cathode. When the electrons strike the focal spot, they are therefore deflected through an x-ray window below the diverted path to the digital sensor. The resultant "effective" focal spot is considerably smaller than the spot on the anode and image quality is improved. In addition, the anode can absorb more heat because it is spread over a larger area of that electrode.

SETUP OF A SIMPLE X-RAY TUBE

A simple x-ray tube consists of a tightly closed housing made of leaded glass (usually Pyrex), a negative terminal or cathode comprised of a tungsten filament wire surrounded by a molybdenum cup, and a positively charged copper anode with a central area made of tungsten. The tungsten filament of the cathode serves as a source of electrons when heated. These electrons are set in motion by the application of an extremely high voltage or electrical potential difference between the cathode and anode. The central area of the anode is called the **focal spot**. At the focal spot, about 1% of the energy generated is changed into x-rays with the remainder dissipated as heat production or infrared radiation in the outer portions of the anode. The anode serves as means of suddenly stopping or decelerating the electrons. Tungsten filaments are used because they have very high melting points and are destroyed.

FUNCTION OF THE CATHODE FOCUSING CUP AND REGULATING ELECTRON FLOW

The focusing cup is a receptacle that surrounds the tungsten filament of the x-ray tube cathode. It is usually made of molybdenum. The main purpose of the focusing cup is to direct the flow of electrons to the anode so that they strike a smaller, more focused area of the anode. Otherwise, the electron beam would spread out more, electrons would strike a larger portion of the anode, and the image would not be very distinct. The speed of electron flow is controlled by the amount of potential difference or voltage between the two electrodes. While there is a maximum voltage or

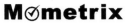

peak (kVp or kilovoltage peak) that can be applied, the actual voltage of individual electrons is variable and usually less that the maximum. A greater gap potential difference will produce a faster electron flow or current, and subsequently x-ray photons with higher frequencies and energies are generated. Higher energy x-rays can penetrate further than those with lower energies.

GENERATION OF ELECTRONS

Electrons are generated in the **tungsten filament of the cathode** of the x-ray tube. When the filament is heated, thermal energy is transmitted to the tungsten and the electrons in its outer orbital shells are stripped off to form a cluster of electrons. This phenomenon is known as thermionic emission. Tungsten does not melt until it reaches 3420 °C, and the filament is typically heated to about two-thirds of that melting point. The rate of electron flow or electrical current measured in milliamperes (mA) is directly related to the applied temperature and the number of electrons pulled off. A typical dental x-ray apparatus generates 7-15 mA.

RESULT WHEN ELECTRONS HIT ANODE AND ITS TARGET IN THE X-RAY TUBE

Electrons streaming from the cathode to the anode in an x-ray tube have what is termed **kinetic or motion-related energy**. When these electrons reach the anode, they are stopped or decelerated. A portion of these electrons hit the tungsten target where the electrons in the shell orbits of the tungsten become excited. This means that these latter electrons temporarily possess higher energy levels, but as they revert to their initial states energy is given off in the form of either infrared radiation (heat) or as x-rays. The small proportion of x-rays generated (less than 1% usually) are redirected in many directions in the tube, and the x-rays that manage to pass through the x-ray window represent the useful beam for imaging and other purposes.

TYPES OF RADIATION

BREMSSTRAHLUNG RADIATION

In an x-ray tube, two types of radiation are produced, Bremsstrahlung and characteristic radiation. Bremsstrahlung (also called Brems or general radiation) is the dominant type of x-ray elicited by dental x-ray equipment. This general radiation represents photons of energy emitted as a result of a deceleration of the high-speed electrons at the tungsten anode target. This occurs in one of two ways. Usually, high-speed electrons streaming from the cathode are attracted to the positively charged nucleus of the tungsten in the anode target. If opposing nuclear forces are stronger, the fast electron is deflected and slowed down near the nucleus, and x-ray photons are emitted. This pattern of attraction followed by deflection, deceleration, and photon emission continues until the electron's energy is depleted. On the other hand, if the high-speed electron actually collides with and penetrates the nucleus, only one discrete photon of x-ray energy is produced.

CHARACTERISTIC RADIATION

Characteristic radiation is a type of x-ray that is generated when a high-energy electron from the cathode ionizes or removes an electron from an inner orbit of the target. A typical x-ray tube has a tungsten target at the anode. If the cathode electrons hit the target with enough energy, an electron in the innermost K shell of the tungsten is initially ejected. Subsequently, an electron from the next L shell moves to occupy the space in the K shell where the electron was pulled off, and a photon of so-called "characteristic radiation" is released. Characteristic radiation represents the disparity between the binding energies in the two orbital shells, and it is always the same for a particular element (tungsten in this case). In an x-ray tube, a photon of characteristic radiation is 59 keV, or the difference between the binding energy of the K shell of tungsten, 70 keV, and the L shell, 11 keV. This type of radiation is only emitted if the potential difference in the tube equals or exceeds the 70 keV binding energy of the K shell.

68

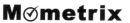

HETEROGENEOUS VS. HOMOGENEOUS RADIATION

Most Brems radiation emitted from a typical dental x-ray tube controlled by alternating current (AC) is **heterogeneous**. This means that the radiation is released in a range of energies and wavelengths. This variety occurs for two reasons. First, the electrons coming from the cathode possess a continuum of speeds due to the AC, and second, most of the electrons gradually lose energy by a series of interactions with different nuclei. Longer wavelength photons either bounce around inside the tube or are filtered out. If the apparatus is designed to convert the AC to direct current (DC), then a more **homogeneous** radiation is effectively emitted, greater penetration of the soft tissues is achieved, and image quality is improved. This is because all the cathode-derived electrons achieve the same voltage difference near the peak applied, and the subsequent radiation emitted is more uniform as well. This also allows for somewhat lower doses of radiation because there are no relatively useless longer wavelength species.

X-RAY GENERATORS

COMPONENTS

A typical x-ray generator used for dental x-rays is comprised of two distinct parts. The first is the **control panel**, which contains all of the controls for parameters such as the exposure time, current selection (mA or milliamperes), potential difference (kVp or kilovoltage peak), and the like plus the actual x-ray emission light. The other part is the **tubehead assembly**, which consists of the x-ray tube and transformers. All of the tubehead assembly is submerged in oil to shield the apparatus and thwart sparks between different components.

SELF-RECTIFICATION OF CURRENT

Most x-ray generators provide electrical energy to the dental x-ray tube in the form of alternating current (AC), typically as 110 or 220 volts in cycles of 60 Hertz (Hz or cycles per second). This means that the electrons generated flow first in one direction from the cathode to the anode by attraction, and then in the other direction. A wavelike pattern is produced in which the current reaches a peak, returns to baseline, and then goes through a trough and returns to baseline when the current is reversed. During this latter trough, current does not stream through the x-ray tube because the anode is already negatively charged. The result is **self-rectification** or effective conversion of the alternating current to unidirectional direct current (DC). In addition, while direction of the AC is changed every 1/120 of a second, the number of useful cycles per second is halved (in other words, 60 Hz).

TRANSFORMERS

Transformers are electromagnetic pieces of equipment that step the voltage potential difference up or down in an efficient manner. They usually consist of an iron core surrounded by two different loops of wire at either end. As the current passes through the core and the first or primary circuit wire, a magnetic field is generated. This in turn sets up a secondary current in the second loop of wire if the magnitude of the magnetic field is shifting, such as when alternating current is applied. The number of times each wire is coiled around the end relative to the other wire determines whether the transformers can step-up or step-down the voltage. The voltage generated in the secondary coil is directly related to the number of coils it possesses relative to the primary wire loop. Some dental x-ray machines have variable autotransformers in which there is only one large coil encircling the iron core. In this case, there are multiple areas where the insulation of the wire has been removed; a metal conductor can be moved to different exposed areas to generate and control the magnitude of the secondary circuit.

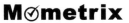

CHANGES FACILITATED BY TRANSFORMERS

In a dental x-ray machine, a filament circuit is activated when the exposure switch is closed. When a step-down transformer is used, the voltage is decreased from the applied 110 or 220 volts in the primary loop to a much lower voltage of about 8-12 volts in the secondary wire. This generates a large current of about 3-6 amperes to heat the cathode filament, which in turn produces more electrons at that location. If a step-up transformer is utilized instead, the applied current is increased in the secondary coil to a very high voltage of about 60-100 kVp. In this case, this extreme potential difference accelerates the movement of the cathode electrons to the anode, while also decreasing the current to about 10-15 milliamperes. Autotransformers are typically used as step-up transformers that can vary the voltage.

IMPACT OF CURRENT ON X-RAY EMISSION SPECTRUM

The current applied using a dental x-ray apparatus is directly related to the number of electrons produced at the cathode filament and the subsequent number of electrons flowing to the electrode. For each heterogeneous x-ray beam, there is a spectrum of emission of x-rays of various wavelengths or photons of different energies. This can be represented in a distribution curve. The setup of a particular machine can shift the proportion of types of x-rays emitted, but in general the beam intensity can be proportionately affected by changes in the current (mA) applied and the electron flow.

RELATIONSHIP BETWEEN EXPOSURE TIME AND CURRENT

More photons of x-ray energy are generated by increasing the exposure time. Often the maximum potential difference (kVp) and current (mA) are preset when doing dental x-rays, and the only variable is the exposure time. In this case, increasing exposure time augments the total energy or intensity. Exposure time can be expressed as either fractions or whole multiples of a second or as the number of impulses of electrical energy applied in a second. Either expression of exposure time can be multiplied by the current applied to give values known as mAs or mAi respectively. In general, the goal is to maintain either mAs or mAi as constant, which can be achieved by changing the current and exposure time in opposition. In other words, if the current is increased the exposure time is decreased and vice versa.

IMPACT OF KILOVOLTAGE ON X-RAY PRODUCTION

Kilovoltage (kVp) is the maximum voltage that occurs across an x-ray tube from the cathode to the anode (although the voltage is not constant). The voltage setting determines the gray scale contrast and quality of the image. X-ray machines may have a fixed setting of between 65 and 75 or may have adjustable settings between 50 and 100. If the kVp is adjusted higher, the velocity of electrons increases and better penetrates, but this decreases contrast in the image, which is then grayer. If the kVp is adjusted lower, the velocity slows and the image has higher contrast, but lacks shades of gray. In both cases, the image suffers, so the ideal settings are usually somewhere in the range of 65-75. The radiation exposure to the patient varies little between 60 and 80. However, settings below 60 increase exposure to the patient, so they are usually avoided.

IMPACT OF KILOVOLTAGE ON WAVELENGTH, FREQUENCY, AND ENERGY

The kilovoltage or potential difference applied influences the number and degree of penetration of the x-rays emitted. Potential differences of between 60 and 65 kVp generate x-rays that do not penetrate much and are termed "soft." These x-rays have relatively long wavelengths and low frequencies and energies. Larger potential differences of usually 85-100 kVp produce x-rays that penetrate either much more or completely and are termed "hard." Here the associated x-ray wavelengths are relatively short, and the energies and frequencies are higher. These differences can

70

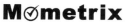
be exploited when performing dental x-rays by using larger voltages in areas that are thick or dense.

X-Ray Beam Intensity

The intensity of an x-ray beam is its total energy emitted per unit area and time. Total energy is the product of two key components, the quantity or number of photons in the beam, and the quality or energy of the specific photons. Area is defined in terms of the cross-sectional space at the point of measurement on the image; this is proportional to the distance from the source which can be controlled. The exposure rate or time can also be regulated by the technician as can the voltage and current applied. Thus, the beam intensity can be calculated as:

$$\text{Intensity} = \frac{(\text{quantity of photons}) \times (\text{quality})}{(\text{cross sectional area}) \times (\text{exposure time})}$$

Radiographic Density

The density is a reading of the relative darkness, blackness, or radiolucency of areas of a dental image. Factors that influence the density of an image include the patients hard and soft tissues, the amount of x-rays generated at the filament circuit, and the speed at which the x-rays travel from the cathode to the anode in the tubehead. Images that are overall light in appearance lack density and can be referred to as low density images. Images that are conversely very dark are said to have high density.

Characteristic Curve

A characteristic curve is an xy-plot of image density (y) versus the logarithm of the exposure time (x). Each type of image has its own characteristic curve depending on where in the mouth the sensor is placed. The plot looks like an elongated S with a bottom or toe part, a long relatively straight-line portion in the middle, and a shoulder at the top. The middle straight-line part of the curve can be defined by its slope, or the change in the density relative to log of relative exposure time (y/x). The straight-line portion is also the zone of correct exposure. Images with steeper slopes provide more contrast than those with shallower slopes.

Impact of Acceptable Exposure Times

The range of acceptable exposure times can also be extrapolated from the characteristic curve by drawing lines from the y density axis in the desired range (for example, about 0.5-2.5); only exposure times falling in that range are diagnostically useful. There is a degree of tolerance or exposure error, termed latitude, inherent in an image that is inversely proportional to its slope and corresponding contrast. In other words, there is little latitude or room for error with high contrast images and vice versa. Kilovoltage applied affects the amount of latitude in the acceptable range of exposure times directly because of its inverse relationship to contrast.

Influencing Variables

Aspects of the actual radiographic exposure are the most important variables that control radiographic density, particularly the product mAs. Milliampere seconds, or mAs, is the multiplication product between the current in milliamperes times the exposure time in seconds. This is important because it directly affects the number of x-rays hitting the and the amount of silver that aggregates. The kilovoltage difference in the x-ray tube is also significant because it controls the wavelength and frequency of the x-rays, and the most penetrating x-rays occur with high voltage and resultant short wavelengths. Density is also inversely related to the square of the distance between the x-ray beam and the sensor.

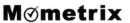

VOLTAGE CHANGES, EXPOSURE TIMES, AND THE ABILITY TO CONTROL DENSITY

When voltage is increased, the intensity of the emitted x-ray increases as well. However, this relationship is more than linear; the factor the voltage is stepped up by must be squared to calculate the intensity. In addition, voltage increases are related to the current produced and ideal exposure time. A particular density or darkness of an image is usually desired. Two schemes are generally followed to achieve this density. One states that the current in milliamperes should be cut in half for every 15% augmentation in voltage. Alternatively, the exposure time must be divided in two for every voltage rise of 15 kVp or doubled for each similar reduction of potential difference.

INVERSE SQUARE LAW IN RELATION TO DEVICE POSITIONING

X-rays generated at the target on the anode are filtered through a collimating device upon leaving the tubehead. Then these rays are usually directed to the patient through the use of a beam- or position-indicating device. The intensity of the x-ray beam when it strikes the sensor in the patient's mouth is related to the distance of the sensor from the tungsten target in the tubehead e by a relationship called the **inverse square law**. This law states that the intensity of the radiation at the level of the sensor is inversely related to the square of the distance between the source of radiation and the sensor. For example, doubling the length of the positioning indicator device cuts down the radiation intensity that strikes the sensor by a factor of 4 (in other words, $2^2 = 4$). This can be compensated for by increasing the exposure time by the same factor of 4.

CONTRAST

LONG-SCALE VS SHORT-SCALE RADIOGRAPHIC CONTRAST

Radiographic contrast is the difference between the densities of extremely dark and light portions of a radiograph. The most important factor controlling contrast is the kilovoltage potential difference in the x-ray tube. Generally, at lower kilovoltages of 60-65 kV, **short-scale contrast** is observed; at these voltages, the x-rays emitted have long wavelengths but lower energy. On the other hand, if higher voltages of 80-90 kV are used, **long-scale contrast** is usually observed. Here the x-rays have shorter wavelengths and greater penetrability, resulting in more gradations of gray.

RELATIONSHIP BETWEEN CONTRAST, DENSITY, AND EXPOSURE TIME

Contrast is theoretically controlled by the kilovoltage applied. The density or darkness of an image is affected by a number of factors. The most important variable is milliampere seconds, but kilovoltage also increases the density. When either exposure time or the mAs product is altered, the image density is affected, but contrast is not, unless the kVp potential difference is also changed. In practice, lower mAs (and exposure times) are usually utilized with the higher voltages producing low or long-scale contrast, and higher values of these parameters are generally used with lower voltages and high or short-scale contrast.

INDICATIONS

Use of long-scale radiographic contrast conditions is generally preferred for radiographs of the periapical areas and bony changes like periodontal or periapical disease. Conditions favoring short-scale radiographic contrast are usually recommended for bitewing images and the illustration of caries or tooth decay. Ideal densities and contrasts are subjective, however. Low voltage, short-scale images, may not show early pathologic alterations. Images with long-scale can identify early changes better, and some clinicians prefer these for caries. The downside of images with long-scale is that they are not as crisp and visually pleasing.

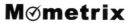

SPATIAL CHARACTERISTICS THAT INFLUENCE THE DETAIL AND DEFINITION OF IMAGES

The central sharp area of a radiographic image is called the **umbra**, and it is surrounded by a blurrier area called the **penumbra**. The less sharp penumbra area can be reduced by decreasing the target area on the anode and the effective focal area. Images are also distorted on radiographs because materials furthest from the sensor will be magnified more than those closer. This distortion can influence the perceived shape of the tooth or other objects as well. These distortions are related to the attempt to visualize three-dimensional objects on the flat plane of a sensor. Detail or definition is also influenced by the distances between the sensor and either the focal point or the object being imaged. Movement of the patient or any equipment or the use of intensifying screens can decrease definition and produce blurriness. Definition is directly related to contrast.

Radiation Protection

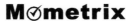

Radiation Physics

BASIC STRUCTURE OF AN ATOM

An atom is the smallest portion into which an element can be divided and still retain its inherent properties. Elements are the simplest units of matter and they cannot be broken down into other substances by chemical reactions. The number of identified elements has changed over time; 118 is the current number. The atom is comprised of a central nucleus containing a set number of positively charged protons and neutral neutrons, which is surrounded by rings or orbits of negatively charged electrons. These electrons stay in orbit because of their electrostatic attraction to the protons. The atomic or Z number is an expression of the number of protons in the atom.

IONIZATION

Ionization is the conversion of an atom from a neutral to either a positive or negative charge. The charge represents the discrepancy between the number of protons in the nucleus and the number of electrons after ionization, and the charged atom is called an ion. If outer orbital shells are unfilled, the atom has a tendency to acquire electrons, and it becomes a negatively charged anion. If electrons are lost, the result is a positively charged atom or cation. X-ray bombardment of an atom conveys energy to the orbital electron; the electron is ejected but forms a loose attraction to the atom termed an ion pair.

FORCES OF ATTRACTION AND BINDING ENERGY FOR ORBITAL ELECTRONS

Electrons circle around the nucleus in up to 7 different paths or shells, which are sequentially lettered from K to Q. Shell K is closest to the nucleus, and shell Q is the theoretical furthest path. Normally, there is equilibrium between the centrifugal and electrostatic forces that enables each electron to stay in orbit. However, electrons in the outer orbital shells are more easily removed from the atom since less work or energy is required to strip the electrons from outer orbital shells than the inner paths. Electrons occupying the external shell are called valence electrons because they are easily removed and can thus establish the atom's chemical properties, including its optical spectrum. Binding energy is the amount of energy needed to extract an electron from its orbit; this parameter is distinctive for each element and each orbital shell.

ELECTRON VOLT AND BINDING ENERGY

An electron volt is a measurement of kinetic or motion-related energy. It is defined as the amount of energy generated by moving an electron through an electrical potential difference of 1 volt. It is often expressed as kiloelectron (keV) or megaelectron (MeV) volts, which are 1000 or 1 million times a single volt. Each shell of an atom has a defined binding energy which is generally expressed in keV. Electrons can be removed from the shell if that binding energy is achieved through bombardment with x-rays or other rays or particles. While loosely held electrons in the outermost paths can be removed by low energy visible light or UV rays, electrons in the closer shells can only be pulled off with higher energy x-rays, gamma rays, or certain particles.

PARTICULATE RADIATIONS

Particulate radiations are small masses that travel linearly at rapid speed and can penetrate matter. Only one type of particulate radiation is neutral in charge, the neutron. All of the other types are electrically charged, and the degree of penetration is generally inversely related to the particle mass. One variety is the alpha particle, a helium nucleus without the associated electrons, which is 2 protons plus 2 neutrons. These particles are emitted from heavy metals and are heavy and highly charged; thus, alpha particles lose energy quickly and do not penetrate matter as well as other types of particulate radiation. The much smaller electrons penetrate tissue and air much more effectively. Electrons are emitted as particulate radiations as either beta particles (negatrons) from

74

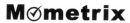

radioactive nuclei or as cathode rays (electrons). Cathode rays are actually flows of orbital electrons that are generated from the filament of an x-ray tube and travel from the cathode to the anode. The nuclei of the hydrogen atom can be sped up and emitted as another form of particulate radiation, a proton, but the mass of these protons is large, and they do not penetrate very effectively.

ELECTROMAGNETIC RADIATION AND DIAGNOSTIC RADIOLOGY

Electromagnetic radiation is energy traveling in space while generating electric and magnetic force fields. There are two types of electromagnetic radiation, **gamma rays** discharged from disintegrating radioactive nuclei, and **x-rays** emitted outside the nucleus without mass or electrical charge. X-rays can travel through tissues further than other forms of radiation without focal localization, making them important for forms of diagnostic radiology including dental radiographs. Particulate radiation like alpha and beta particles or the electromagnetic gamma rays are more useful in nuclear medicine treatments.

PARTICLE CONCEPTS OF ELECTROMAGNETIC RADIATION

In addition to spreading in a wave-like pattern, x-rays and other narrow wavelength, high frequency electromagnetic radiations can act like particles. Distinct parcels of energy called quanta or photons are disseminated by these types of radiations. These energy bundles do not have mass. If the frequency of the wavelength is increased (in other words, the wavelength is shortened), the energy of the photon is increased proportionately. If the energy level reaches or exceeds 15 electron volts, orbital electrons of atoms can be pulled off. This is known as ionization, and the associated types of rays are considered to be ionizing radiation. Examples of this type of radiation include not only x-rays but gamma rays and certain types of ultraviolet rays.

WAVE PROPAGATION

Electromagnetic radiations, including x-rays, disseminate energy in **wave-like patterns**. The speed of dissemination of these rays is equivalent to the speed of light, which is defined as either 186,000 miles per second or 3×10^8 miles per second. Electromagnetic waves are distinguished by the fact that they do not require a medium to pass through; instead, they can spread in a vacuum. X-rays and other waves are characterized by the interrelated constant speed of light (often shown as the letter c) and the variables of wavelength and frequency. Wavelength is the length between the same phase in adjoining waves, and it is usually expressed in meters or the Greek letter lambda (λ). Frequency is the number of wave cycles occurring per second, it is measured in hertz, and it can be represented by the Greek letter nu (ν). The relationship between these can be expressed as $c = \lambda\nu$.

ELECTROMAGNETIC SPECTRUM

The electromagnetic spectrum is the entire range of electromagnetic types of radiation. It is defined by the classification of the type of radiation and its associated wavelength range. The wavelength differences represented in the spectrum are quite large. The **long wavelength**, **low frequency** forms include alternating current, radio waves, television, and radar. These wave cycles range from about 10^{12} meters down to several meters. Infrared, visible, and ultraviolet light have **mid-range wavelengths**. Ionizing radiations such as gamma rays and x-rays have extremely **short wavelengths** and are thus often represented in nanometers (nm), or 10^{-9} meters. The effective wavelengths for medical or dental x-rays are about 0.01–0.05 nanometers. Another unit of measurement is the angstrom unit (A) which is equivalent to a tenth of a nanometer.

CHARACTERISTIC X-RAYS AND THEIR USE IN DENTISTRY AND MEDICINE

X-rays are extremely short wavelength electromagnetic radiations that travel at the speed of light. They have no mass. They disseminate in wave-like patterns in a straight line, but they can be

75

redirected into other linear paths. X-ray beams spread out with increasing distance from the source. X-rays can go through materials that are impenetrable by longer wavelength sources. Certain materials such as digitized sensors can selectively absorb x-rays. X-rays can ionize substances including gases; this property is utilized in ionization chambers. X-rays can also induce changes in biological materials such as human tissues, and this is the basis for their utility in therapeutic radiology.

PRIMARY VS. SECONDARY RADIATION

Primary radiation is the central x-ray beam that leaves the tubehead and is sometimes referred to as the useful x-ray beam because it is responsible for production of the radiographic image. This type of radiation is the most penetrating.

Secondary radiation occurs when the primary radiation interacts with the tissue. When x-rays deflect as they interact with tissue, this form of secondary radiation is referred to as **scatter radiation**. Scatter radiation can go in all directions and poses a risk to both the patient and the operator who may be exposed, so the operator must be at least 6 feet from the patient or behind adequate shielding. Types of scatter radiation include:

- **Compton**: Collision with an electron causes the photon to lose energy and change path, and ionization occurs. Compton scatter is responsible for about 62% of scatter radiation.
- **Photoelectric**: When an x-ray photon is absorbed, an inner shell electron is ejected, and then another electron releases a characteristic photon to fill that void. The photoelectric scatter is responsible for about 30% of scatter radiation.
- **Coherent**: Also called Thompson or unmodified scattering, this collision alters the photon path, but no ionization occurs. Coherent scatter is responsible for about 8% of scatter radiation.

THE PHOTOELECTRIC EFFECT

X-rays can be taken into matter and tissues when the two interact, a process called **photoelectric absorption**. This generally happens when the energy level of the photon is slightly greater than the binding energy of the material's K or innermost orbital shell. The x-ray is absorbed into and transfers its energy to the orbital electron, which is expelled and taken in by another atom. Atoms with higher atomic numbers tend to absorb x-rays more readily. Photoelectric absorption is more prevalent with high frequency, low wavelength x-rays or when the interacting material is thick or dense. This phenomenon has also been classified as **characteristic radiation**; the energies to expel the K shell electron and replace it with an L shell electron are both predetermined. The energy difference defines the energy of the resultant x-ray

FOGGED IMAGES

Fogged images, or images with an undesired darkness, can result when radiation that has been scattered interacts with the sensor. There are two ways in which this scatter of radiation can occur:

- A small portion of the radiation can undergo **Thompson scattering**, also known as unmodified or coherent scattering. In this case, lower energy photons change direction when they encounter matter but little else occurs.

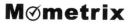

- Another phenomenon called Compton or **incoherent** is more prevalent, and it is a potentially greater problem for x-ray interpretation. Here higher energy x-rays expel outermost orbital electrons upon interaction with matter; this results in a positively charged atom loosely coupled to a negatively charged Compton or recoil electron. The origin photon changes direction and undergoes subsequent similar interactions and directional changes. If the angle of change is small, most of the intensity of the photon remains, and it can easily arrive at the sensor as fog.

The majority of dental x-ray photons experience this type of scattering, so manipulations are usually necessary to reduce it. These manipulations can include use of rectangular collimators and changing other parameters to shorten exposure time.

Radiation Protection

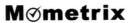

Radiation Biology

EFFECTS OF X-RADIATION ON ATOMS AND MOLECULES

When an x-ray photon comes in contact with an atom or molecule, the molecular structure is changed. In some cases, the energy from the photon causes orbital electrons in the atom to vibrate or become excited. The result is either release of light and heat or the actual disruption of molecular bonds. If the energy of the x-ray is enough to expel the orbital electron from the atom, a second phenomenon called **ionization** occurs. In this case, an electron can be ejected or loosely bound to form an ion pair with the now positively charged atom. If molecular bonds are broken, molecules act differently and cell function can be disrupted.

RADIOLYSIS

Radiolysis is the breakdown of chemicals into smaller components by x-rays or other radiation. The term usually refers to the interface of this radiation with water molecules because water makes up about 80% of the body. Subsequently, an ion pair of the positively charged water and a free electron or radical is created. The term free radical can describe any molecule containing an unpaired electron, though, and all of these are very chemically reactive and able to destroy life components like deoxyribonucleic acid, DNA, and adenosine triphosphate, ATP. For example, two hydroxyl (*OH) radicals can combine to form a harmful substance called hydrogen peroxide (H_2O_2).

THEORY OF ACCUMULATIVE EFFECT OF RADIATION

It has been theorized that the biological effects of radiation are cumulative. That means that the untoward effects of radiation exposure accumulate in increments with each contact. The consensus opinion is also that low-dose ionizing radiation (like that used in dentistry) has a non-threshold, linear type of dose-response curve. The concept of accumulative effect is premised upon the idea that repair after radiation exposure is never complete. This cumulative effect eventually can lead to malignancies, birth defects, aging, and other diseases. Damaging effects are not evident until a certain amount of time, called the latent period, has elapsed between exposure and documented consequences. The potential effects of the radiation are dependent on a number of host factors and radiation parameters.

TYPES OF EFFECTS THAT RADIATION HAS ON BIOLOGICAL MATERIALS

Radiation can affect biological materials either directly or indirectly. When radiation interacts directly with biologically active materials, the destruction is a direct effect. The most significant direct effect is the breakdown of DNA in the nucleus of the cell, which prevents further cell processes including replication resulting in cell death. Radiation can have a direct destructive effect on other important molecules like proteins and ribonucleic acid (RNA) as well. Ionizing radiation can also act indirectly by producing free radicals that later either react with life-sustaining molecules or form intermediate toxic substances that affect biological materials. The effects of radiation can be cell damage or in rare instances malignant changes.

RESPONSES OF SOMATIC AND GENETIC TISSUES TO RADIATION DOSES

When somatic tissues are exposed to radiation, changes do not occur until a particular threshold radiation dose is reached. The relationship between the radiation dose and subsequent tissue damage is not linear but looks like a curve on a two-dimensional plot. These effects do not affect the genetic makeup of the individual. Rather they include effects like sunburn or other skin reddening, hair loss, development of cataracts on the eye, or sterility.

On the other hand, genetic changes such as those occurring in reproductive tissues involve mutations in the DNA that can be passed on to the next generation or cause malignancies. In these

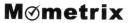

tissues, the relationship between the amount of radiation exposure and number of mutations is linear. These genetic tissues do not need a threshold dose of radiation before mutations occur (termed non-threshold). There are other cellular mechanisms that can moderate the effects of radiation such as repair of DNA and other structures, destruction of the cell by other cells called phagocytes, and stimulation of the immune system.

REASON FOR INCREASED SUSCEPTIBILITY TO THE EFFECTS OF RADIATION

Most mammals, including humans, are more susceptible to the effects of radiation than other species. It is difficult to pinpoint why certain individual human beings are more sensitive to radiation damage than others. However, it has been demonstrated that certain human organs and tissues are more radiosensitive than others. The most sensitive cell types are those that divide very rapidly, in particular tissues involved with blood formation (like bone marrow) or reproduction (such as the ovary) or those cells that are already malignant; cells in these categories are killed relatively easily by exposure to radiation. The least sensitive cell types, termed radioresistant cells, are those that do not divide often, such as muscle and nerve cells.

GREATEST BIOLOGICAL RISKS FROM DENTAL RADIATION EXPOSURE

The greatest biological risks from dental radiation exposure are the possible development of two types of **malignancies**: leukemia and thyroid cancer. Dental x-rays augment the natural probability that an individual may develop these cancers by increased exposure. Leukemia is cancer of the bone marrow, which is involved in blood cell production. Since about 10% of the body's bone marrow is in the skull region, and about a tenth of that is located in the actual mandible, dental radiography does slightly increase the probability of leukemia. The thyroid gland, the endocrine gland at the base of the neck, is close enough to the region typically irradiated during dental x-rays to be subject to scatter radiation. There are thyroid collars that can be worn by the patient to eliminate about half of the already low dose of scatter radiation.

AREAS OF BODY TO AVOID DURING DENTAL RADIOGRAPHY

Genetic abnormalities and malignancies can result from radiation exposure. For dental radiography, the gonads and reproductive systems of patients should always be shielded to prevent these abnormalities or fetal congenital defects. Exposure to the bone marrow, thyroid gland, or unnecessary areas of skin should be avoided as well because of the possibility of development of leukemia or other malignancies. In addition, cataract development has been associated with exposure of the lens of the eye to radiation so that area should be avoided as well.

TRANSMISSION OF RADIATION EFFECTS TO THE NEXT GENERATION

In general, the changes induced by radiation exposure are only transmitted to the next generation when these effects occur in genetic or reproductive tissues. In these types of tissues, the radiation actually causes changes in the genetic material, and these changes are then passed on to the next generation. On the other hand, all other cell types are termed somatic; they include skin, connective tissues, nerves and a wide variety of other tissues and organs. When somatic tissues are changed by radiation exposure, these changes are not transmitted to the progeny.

WHY DENTAL RADIOGRAPHY IS CONSIDERED RELATIVELY BENIGN

There are various types of radiation. The radiation from dental x-rays is sparsely ionizing. This means that the energy they transfer is dispersed and these x-rays are said to have a low linear energy transfer (LET). Other types of radiation, in particular alpha particles, have a higher LET, deposit the energy in more discrete bundles, and have a considerably higher potential for biological damage. In addition, very small quantities of radiation are used for dental radiographs, most of the x-rays do not reach internal tissues because they are absorbed by outer layers of the skin, and only

Radiation Protection

79

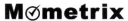

small areas of the head and neck are generally exposed. Short but intense acute exposure to radiation is generally more damaging than prolonged but smaller chronic exposure. Dental radiography might be considered chronic exposure because of its low level, repetitive nature.

MINIMIZING BIOLOGICAL RISKS

Most dental offices utilize leaded torso aprons for their patients while taking dental images, thus virtually eliminating whole body and specifically reproductive organ exposure. These aprons are especially important as preventive measures for pregnant females to reduce the possibility of fetal congenital defects. There are few documented studies about the effects of radiation on genetic changes in reproductive organs and subsequent transmission to children. Even without aprons, the uterus and fetus receive only minor secondary radiation. Other possible risks like cataract development require a threshold dose of radiation before untoward effects are observed. At the exposure levels of typical dental x-rays, the risk is very small because the values are far below the threshold.

MEASUREMENT SYSTEMS FOR RADIATION DOSE

The traditional **units of measurement** for radiation dose were the **roentgen** or **R**, **rad**, and **rem**. All of these terms are equivalent, and measurements of dosage can be expressed with the smaller units of milliroentgens (mR), millirads (mrad), or millirems (mrem). While these units are still often used, there is also a newer **SI classification system**. In the SI system, units are expressed in gray (Gy) or sievert (Sv) units as well as centigray or cGy and milligray or mGy. The relationship between the two systems is 1 gray per 100 rads. These are all units of dose, or the amount of energy from the x-ray that is taken in per mass unit of tissue. For example, the gray unit represents the number of Joules of energy absorbed per kilogram of tissue. Dose absorbed is a more important parameter than exposure because it corresponds to potential biological destruction.

RADIATION EXPOSURE VS. RADIATION DOSE

Radiation exposure represents the number of photons producing a particular electrical charge in a volume of air. Originally, exposure was measured by converting the number of roentgen units, which quantified the number of ion pairs per cubic centimeter of air, into the electrical charge produced, which was expressed in coulombs or C. Today, exposure is expressed in exposure units, which are defined as one coulomb per kilogram of air. Exposure does not necessarily reflect the actual radiation dose delivered to tissues, and this dosage is highly dependent on a number of factors like tissue density and host response. The modern dose unit is the SI unit or gray. Dose was previously (and still is sometimes) expressed in rad; 1 rad is equivalent to 100 erg (a measurement of energy as well) absorbed per gram of tissue.

DOSE EQUIVALENTS
MODELS OF DOSE EQUIVALENTS

Different types of radiation can produce varying amounts of biological damage with the same dose. X-rays, beta particles, and gamma rays all possess the least potential for destruction. They have been assigned a quality factor (QF) of 1. Other more damaging types of radiation have been assigned higher QFs, which represent their relative destructive power. The concept of dose equivalents (H) expresses the relative destructive effects of different radiation types in Sieverts or mSv by multiplying the dose (D) in Gy by the assigned quality factor (QF). All types of radiation (including x-rays) with a QF of 1 have equal doses and dose equivalents so the number of Gy and Sv are the same. For more destructive types of radiation like neutrons or alpha particles, the number of dose equivalents (Sv) is larger than the dose absorbed by a factor, the QF.

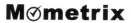

EFFECTIVE DOSE EQUIVALENTS

The risk of development of genetic defects or cancer from radiation exposure is dependent on the location and breadth of exposure in addition to the number of dose equivalents absorbed. The reason is that certain tissues are more susceptible to damaging biological effects and malignancy, in particular reproductive and blood-forming tissues and certain organs like the breast. Therefore, the concept of effective dose equivalents defines the relative destructive power based on area of exposure. In dentistry for example, a bitewing or panoramic radiograph exposes the patient to very low effective dose equivalents, while a full-mouth intraoral set that includes multiple images multiplies this effective dose. X-rays used in other settings such as nuclear medicine expose the patient to beams in much larger areas of the body including potential genetic targets and deliver much higher effective doses. They are often termed whole body exposures.

Radiation Protection

81

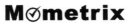

Patient/Operator Exposure to Radiation and Radiation Safety

IMPACT OF FILTRATION, SHIELDING, COLLIMATION AND PID LENGTH

Factors influencing radiation safety include the following:

Filtration	Aluminum filter placed at cone base covers the opening through which the x-ray beam travels to absorb low-energy photons and allow-high energy photons to pass through, reducing exposure. Filters range from a minimum of 1.5 mm for machines with kVp below 70, to 2.5 mm for machines with kVp above 70.
Shielding	Lead and lead-equivalent shielding devices, such as thyroid collars and aprons, reduce exposure.
Collimation	Lead diaphragm restricts x-ray beam to conform to the size and shape of the image receptor in order to decrease scatter radiation and patient exposure. The lead collimator with a round or rectangular opening limits the beam size to ≤2.75 inches.
PID [cone] length	The length of the position indicating device (PID) or cone, which is lead lined, affects the target-receptor distance. While cylindrical and rectangular PIDS do not spread scatter radiation, the cone-shaped PIDs do. A short cone (8 inch) requires less radiation but results in more scatter radiation. A long cone requires 4 times more radiation.

REGULATING BODIES FOR RADIATION HEALTH AND SAFETY

NATIONAL ORGANIZATIONS

There are a number of bodies in the United States and internationally that make recommendations on, or actually govern, radiation health and safety. In the United States, a subsidiary of the Food and Drug Administration (FDA), the Center for Devices and Radiological Health (CDRH) controls the manufacture of x-ray machines and other devices emitting radiation. Occupational exposure guidelines are established by the Nuclear Regulatory Commission (NRC), the Occupational Safety and Health Administration (OSHA), or indirectly by the Environmental Protection Agency (EPA) as well. There are also several nationally-based organizations that make recommendations related to radiation health and safety including the Biological Effects of Ionizing Radiation Committee (BEIR) operating under the National Academy of Sciences and the National Council on Radiological Protection and Measurement (NCRP). Every state has a Bureau of Radiation Safety that regulates radiation procedures locally.

INTERNATIONAL ORGANIZATIONS

Several international organizations keep abreast of radiation biology research and make recommendations based on current information. These bodies include the United Nations Scientific Committee on the Effects of Atomic Radiation (UNSCEAR) and the International Commission of Radiological Protection (ICRP). There is also an official worldwide group that proposes standards for radiological units of measurement called the International Commission on Radiation Units and Measurements (ICRU).

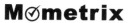

OSHA HAZARD COMMUNICATION STANDARDS FOR CHEMICAL AGENTS

According to the OSHA Hazard Communication Standards (HCS) regarding chemical agents, employees must have access to hazard information associated with their workplace. OSHA's minimum requirements include:

- **Hazard communication program**: A document that outlines the employer's responsibilities, including a list of hazardous chemical and notation of where the list and safety data sheets (SDSs) will be maintained. It should include warning labeling requirements, a description of training courses, and methods of informing contractors of hazards
- List of any hazardous chemicals used in the workplace.
- **Copies of manufacturers' SDSs** for every chemical used in the workplace.
- **Employee training**: This should include summary of OSHA HCS, detection methods, health hazards, signs/symptoms of exposure, good practices, need for personal protective equipment, emergency procedures for spills or exposures, first aid measures for exposures, locations of chemical lists and SDSs, explanation of SDSs, labeling system utilized, and where to obtain additional information.

REGULATIONS GOVERNING DENTAL EQUIPMENT AND LICENSURE REQUIREMENTS

Use of various types of dental equipment must meet official federal performance standards. Radiation standards are generally also established locally by the city, county, and state. In particular, radiation inspections are usually required 2 or 3 times a year. In terms of professional licensure for radiation use, states generally set their own guidelines. A dental hygienist is a licensed specialist, but additional certification in radiography may or may not be obligatory. A dental assistant may be expected to take an examination related to radiology if they take radiographs. For both types of professionals, some states only require general supervision by or presence of a dentist.

AMERICAN DENTAL ASSOCIATION (ADA) GUIDELINES
NEW PATIENTS

Exposure to radiation through use of dental radiographs is a clinical judgment call, and it is not always necessary every dental visit. All radiographic exams should be individualized for new patients. Children who do not have permanent teeth yet may not require dental images, but if the dentist cannot inspect certain areas of the mouth, some periapical, occlusal, or posterior bitewing views might be taken. After their permanent teeth begin to erupt, these types of radiographs plus panoramic views are usually taken. For adolescents or adults with complete or at least partial dentition, posterior bitewings plus panoramic and/or some periapical views are typically done. If history or evidence of dental disease is present, a full mouth radiograph is usually taken. The diagnostic plan for edentulous or toothless adults should be very individualized based on clinical criteria.

RETURNING PATIENTS

The dentist should exercise clinical judgment before radiographs are done on returning patients. If the patient had previous caries or appears to be at risk for development of decay, then posterior bitewing radiographs are usually indicated at 6- to 12-month intervals for children and adolescents and up to 18-month intervals for adults. If caries development or predilection was not previously observed, the period between bitewing x-rays can be increased up to 2 years for children and 3 years for adolescents and adults. If periodontal disease is observed, the dentist should decide what radiographs need to be taken, but typically they include selected bitewing or periapical views. Generally toothless adults do not need to have radiographs done.

PATIENT PROTECTION FROM UNNECESSARY X-RAY EXPOSURE

Unnecessary x-ray exposure may result from:

- Improper positioning of the patient and/or equipment
- An x-ray beam that is larger than necessary, exposing additional tissue
- Use of a cylindrical collimator with rectangular image receptor, allowing increased scatter radiation
- Use of long cone rather than short increases radiation exposure
- Inadequate use and/or placement of body shielding
- Multiple unnecessary exposures
- Too frequent dental x-ray screening
- Inadequate training of operator in proper techniques
- Use of standard radiography rather than digital, which has less radiation exposure
- Use of bisecting method for the x-ray beam rather than parallel, increasing exposure to the eye and thyroid gland
- Short target-receptor distance (8 inches) with parallel method increases tissue exposed to radiation

MAXIMUM PERMISSIBLE DOSE

MPD is the abbreviation for maximum permissible dose of radiation a person is permitted to receive from artificial causes of radiation. The MPD is generally a recommendation of the NCRP, which acquires legal status through local or federal legislation. The MPD is generally higher for groups that are occupationally exposed like dentists and their assistants than for staff members or the general public, who are said to be non-occupationally exposed. A radiation worker who is pregnant is allowed to receive approximately the same lower level of dosage permitted for those non-occupationally exposed. These limits are not imposed for dental or medical procedures that may utilize radiation for patient benefit.

CURRENT RECOMMENDATIONS

At present, the annual effective MPD dose for radiation workers is a whole-body dose of 50 mSv, with higher amounts to certain body parts up to 750 mSv on the hands. Workers falling into this category are permitted to receive a cumulative lifetime exposure of 10 times their age in years (for example, 500 mSv for an individual 50 years of age). The public or anyone non-occupationally exposed should receive only 1-5 mSv, depending on whether their exposure is continuous (as in several dental x-rays) or infrequent. Doses to specific areas like the lens of the eye can approach 150 mSv. Anyone training in the dental profession who is younger than 18 years old is subject to these limits as well. A pregnant woman should never receive more than 0.5 mSv a month up to a maximum of 5 mSv during the time she carries the child. In practice, the recommendation is to permit "as low as reasonably achievable" (ALARA) radiation, which is ideally lower than imposed MPD.

SOURCES OF BACKGROUND RADIATION

The environment exposes individuals to background radiation. In the United States, this background level is about 3 mSv with the major type of exposure being from radon gas. In some other countries, the background radiation levels have been documented to be up to 13 times higher than in the United States without demonstrable changes in the population rate of malignancies or birth defects. Areas of high altitude have a slightly higher background level of radiation. Typically, the effective dose of ionizing radiation that an individual in the U. S. receives from dental imaging is only about 0.1 percent of their total radiation received. Medical diagnostic procedures on average

84

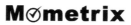

account for much greater doses experienced than those with dental imaging. Nevertheless, background radiation undoubtedly supplies the greatest dosage, more than 80% of the total in the US. Total dosage in the U. S. is projected to be about 4.4 mSv per person.

LOWERING RADIATION DOSAGE EXPOSURE DURING DENTAL RADIOGRAPHY

MANAGING X-RAY MACHINE PARAMETERS

Lowering radiation exposure through x-ray machine adjustment can be achieved by using the higher potential difference in the tube (though no greater than 90 kVp) and/or filtering out the longer wavelength x-rays. The filtration is commonly accomplished by insertion of an aluminum filter. Legislation also dictates that the cross-sectional area of the beam can be no greater than 7 centimeters in diameter if round. Therefore, x-ray machines usually have diaphragms or collimators that restrict the beam area. Rectangular is superior to round collimation because it lessens the exposed area, reduces scatter-induced fogging, and thus produces a better image as well. Selection of a longer 16-inch beam indicating device that is lined with lead restricts radiation dosage most effectively. Use of machines with integrated electronic timers provides more precision. In addition, some newer machines have generators that can convert AC to DC and thus produce a constant wavelength beam.

REDUCING DOSAGE TO THE PATIENT OUTSIDE OF THE X-RAY MACHINE

Potential whole-body and thyroid irradiation can be drastically reduced through the use of leaded torso aprons and thyroid shields. Devices such as the RINN XCP that hold the sensor in place during exposure should be used for many reasons including elimination of finger exposure and more precise placement of the sensor relative to the teeth and the positioning device.

OPERATOR X-RADIATION EXPOSURE

SOURCES OF X-RADIATION TO OPERATORS AND OTHER STAFF

Sources of x-radiation to operators/other staff while exposing image receptors include:

- **Secondary radiation** from standing too close to source of radiation or not being properly shielded. Operator should be at least 6 feet from source or behind shielding.
- Exposure to **primary radiation** if standing in the direct path of the beam or outside of the safe zone (90–135° to the primary beam).
- **Size of x-ray field exceeds that of the image receptor**, allowing increased scatter radiation.
- **Malfunctioning** or **improperly maintained** equipment.
- **Holding the receptor in place in the patient's mouth** or the PID, especially without a device holding the sensor in place.

MONITORING OPERATOR X-RADIATION EXPOSURE

Techniques for monitoring individual x-radiation exposure include:

- Keeping accurate record of radiographic imaging, including frequency and number of images. Patient dosage information should be included in their dental health record when available.
- Avoiding unnecessary or too frequent imaging.

85

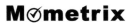

- Wearing a radiation dosimeter (operators): Dosimeter badges contain film, powder, or a lithium fluoride crystal that is sensitive to radiation. The body badges should be placed on the body (attached to clothing) between the neck and waist. Ring badges are also available and used on the hand most likely to come in closest contact to radiation and under gloves. These badges are for occupational use only and should not be worn when receiving x-rays.
- Utilizing an area radiation dosimeter if there are concerns about x-radiation exposure.

REDUCING OCCUPATIONAL RADIATION EXPOSURE

The dental technician or other personnel operating a dental x-ray machine must stand in a position that shields them from the useful x-ray beam as well as potential radiation leakage from the tubehead or scatter from interaction with the patient. In general, this means that dental professionals need to position themselves at least 6 feet away from the patient and at an angle of 90–135° relative to the x-ray beam. If this is impossible, then the operator must wear a leaded protective barrier or stand behind a wall that is dense and deep enough (such as drywall) to absorb the radiation. Other office personnel should be located outside the wall. Radiation exposure to occupationally as well as non-occupationally exposed employees is usually monitored with a dosimeter badge. Individuals wear the dosimeter, which consists of a lithium fluoride crystal, and periodically a dosimetry monitoring service uses the badge to quantify the person's radiation exposure. The badge should be worn in the neck, chest, or hip area.

DETERMINING PROTECTIVE BARRIERS FOR RADIATION PROTECTION

A guide number for protective barriers or walls can be calculated as the product of the workload (W) times the use factor (U) times the occupancy factor (T). Workload is expressed in milliampere minutes per week the machine is used, the use factor is determined by the type of surface (wall versus floor or ceiling) and its orientation to the main x-ray beam, and the occupancy factor reflects the percentage of time the individual remains behind the barrier. Thus, the U for walls is $\frac{1}{4}$, much greater than the U for walls or ceilings which is $\frac{1}{16}$. Similarly, the occupancy for regular office personnel right behind the barrier is 1 while the T for individuals in other areas is much less. Concrete, cinder block, and thick drywall are generally acceptable construction materials.

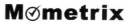

Protocols for Informed Consent and X-Ray Machine Malfunction

INFORMED CONSENT

Dental and medical professionals must obtain informed consent from the patient or their representative (such as the parent or guardian) before initiating procedures. Informed consent involves a complete explanation or full disclosure of the process including its rationale, its benefits, and the possible negative consequences. In the dental office, informed consent should be obtained before performing radiography. If informed consent is denied, the radiograph cannot be taken and an essential part of the diagnostic process is lost.

RESPONDEAT SUPERIOR

The concept of *respondeat superior* is a legal doctrine placing professional and legal liability with the supervising professional. In other words, in a dental practice, the dentist accepts responsibility for the actions of other professionals like dental hygienists or assistants. A hygienist or an assistant under the employ of the dentist is not ultimately responsible, but they could be expected to accept some of the financial burden if found negligent. Therefore, liability insurance is still necessary. An independent contractor can be found responsible and can be sued. In addition, negative input in the office setting can be used as legal evidence of negligence.

DENTAL RECORDS AND OWNERSHIP/RETENTION PARAMETERS

Dental records including radiographs are legal documents. Therefore, dates, number and types of radiographic procedures must be immediately entered. The radiographs themselves must also be tagged, dated, and securely fastened to the chart. All parts of the record are confidential and are considered to be owned by the dentist. The latter means that the dentist is not allowed to give the radiographs to the patient or insurance company, although rules pertaining to distribution of duplicates vary by locality. The minimum period for record retention is 6 or 7 years (depending on local legislation) after the individual stops their association with the dental office.

PROTOCOLS FOR SUSPECTED X-RAY MACHINE MALFUNCTION

Various protocols exist for suspected digital equipment malfunction:

- **Digital x-ray equipment**: Begin by checking the guides for both hardware and software for troubleshooting advice. Items that can be easily assessed before calling for technical support include:
  - USB ports: Try connecting other devices to see if the port is functioning.
  - USB cables: Try switching cables.
  - Interface box: Switch interfaces boxes with one from another room if available to determine if the first is malfunctioning.

If the problem cannot be easily identified and remedied, the machine must be removed from service until it can be repaired.

Chapter Quiz

Ready to see how well you retained what you just read? Scan the QR code to go directly to the chapter quiz interface for this study guide. If you're using a computer, simply visit the bonus page at **mometrix.com/bonus948/danbrhs** and click the Chapter Quizzes link.

Infection Prevention and Control

Transform passive reading into active learning! After immersing yourself in this chapter, put your comprehension to the test by taking a quiz. The insights you gained will stay with you longer this way. Scan the QR code to go directly to the chapter quiz interface for this study guide. If you're using a computer, simply visit the bonus page at **mometrix.com/bonus948/danbrhs** and click the Chapter Quizzes link.

Standard Precautions for Equipment and Supplies

DEFINING SURFACES BASED ON LEVEL OF REQUIRED DECONTAMINATION

A classification system originally developed by E. H. Spaulding breaks down the level of decontamination required for infected objects. In dental radiology, theoretically none of the apparatus or equipment used falls into the highest **critical category**. This classification includes contact with blood products or breaching of tissue, and equipment must either be sterilized or disposed of. Most equipment used in oral and maxillofacial radiology falls into the **semicritical category** because it is in contact with mucous membranes but does not penetrate the tissues. While sterilization procedures are preferred for semicritical items, high-level disinfection measures or barriers can be used. Equipment employed in panoramic or extraoral radiography often falls into the **noncritical category** because while it may come into contact with intact skin, it generally does not touch mucous membranes or saliva, nor does it breach the surrounding tissue. Noncritical items as well as environmental surfaces that the patient does not touch should be sanitized, disinfected with mid-range level products, or protected by barriers.

SOURCES OF CONTAMINATION OF DENTAL PROCESSING SOLUTIONS

The panoramic machine can become contaminated by direct patient contact with the bite block. If the bite block is wrapped with a plastic barrier, then the wrapping should be properly discarded after use. The bite block should be placed in a container and decontaminated after each use. Apparatus involved with panoramic and extraoral imaging should be periodically disinfected as well.

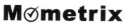

Standard Precautions for Patients and Operators

UNIVERSAL PRECAUTIONS

Universal precautions are a set of safety measures employed in any setting where personnel or patients might be exposed to pathogens that can be transmitted via the blood or saliva. Viruses such as various types of hepatitis (particularly types B and C) and human immunodeficiency virus (HIV) as well as many infectious bacteria are conveyed by blood or saliva. Dental professionals rarely deal with the patient's blood, but they do regularly come into contact with saliva. OSHA has developed the Bloodborne Pathogen (BBP) Rule, and this federal agency can fine medical or dental facilities that do not adhere to the rules. Most states have a State Board of Dental Examiners (BDE) that also enforces guidelines set up by OSHA and other agencies like the American Dental Association (ADA) and the Centers for Disease Control (CDC). The dental healthcare worker must abide by these rules, but responsibility rests with the employer.

PERSONAL PROTECTIVE EQUIPMENT

Personal protective equipment includes impermeable gowns, masks, disposable gloves, and protective eyewear. All of these are usually worn by healthcare workers in many medical settings and in dentistry if the patient is possibly infectious. Examples of the latter include presence of any respiratory infection like a cold or evidence of coughing and possible discharge of fluid aerosols. Since the outbreak of the COVID-19 pandemic, dental radiology personnel are recommended to wear a surgical mask in addition to gloves during all patient contact.

ANTIBIOTIC USE IN SPECIFIC PATIENTS AND DENTAL PERSONNEL IMMUNIZATION

In dentistry, there is a small risk of exposure to blood products. Any invasive treatment could theoretically cause bleeding in the patient. While dental radiography is usually not invasive, the patient typically undergoes other oral probing by the dentist at the same visit. Therefore, a patient may be pre-medicated with **antibiotics** prior to an oral procedure, particularly if they have a history of certain cardiac diseases or artificial joint replacement.

Dental personnel should be **immunized** against tetanus, influenza, varicella, and hepatitis B virus (HBV) because of their potential exposure to infectious blood products.

INFECTION CONTROL PROCEDURES
PANORAMIC RADIOGRAPHY

Panoramic radiography is not invasive. The technician can perform the technique with clean, ungloved hands and theoretically does not need any personal protective equipment during the procedure. The patient should wear a leaded apron, however. The bite guide should either be disposable or can be covered with a plastic bag. Patient cooperation is required because they should use an antibacterial mouthwash and perform the actual placement and removal of the bite block or its covering. After the radiography is performed, equipment that was touched by the patient such as rests or guides should be cleaned.

DIGITAL IMAGING EQUIPMENT STERILIZATION

None of the detectors used with digital processes can be sterilized using heat, and cold chemical methods of sterilization are impractical as well. Infection control procedures for digital imaging with charge coupled devices or CMOS sensors are similar. For both, two layers of plastic barriers are used, a sleeve and an additional finger wrapper. For phosphor (PSP) apparatuses, the primary infection control procedure is the placement of the plate in some type of commercially-available barrier envelope before exposure. The plate is kept bagged until before it is placed in the scanner.

Infection Prevention and Control

AFTER TAKING X-RAYS

For dental radiation procedures, all of the contaminated disposables like gloves, paper towels, and plastic barriers are not defined as infectious materials and can therefore be thrown out in the regular waste. Most other exposed equipment does need to be cleaned or in some cases sterilized. In particular, contaminated sensor holders such as the RINN XCP must initially be put into temporary solutions and later be subjected to other procedures that decontaminate and sterilize them. For sterilization, these items can be put in bags with other contaminated dental equipment and then the bags are autoclaved (steam sterilized) or put in a dry-heat oven. Plastic wrap covering switches or other parts of the x-ray machine can be replaced or sprayed or swabbed with a disinfectant, and lead aprons and collars should be disinfected as well. A clean pair of gloves should be worn during these procedures. Gowns or protective eyewear, if worn, should be regularly laundered or disinfected respectively.

Chapter Quiz

Ready to see how well you retained what you just read? Scan the QR code to go directly to the chapter quiz interface for this study guide. If you're using a computer, simply visit the bonus page at **mometrix.com/bonus948/danbrhs** and click the Chapter Quizzes link.

DANB Practice Test

Want to take this practice test in an online interactive format?
Check out the bonus page, which includes interactive practice questions and much more: **mometrix.com/bonus948/danbrhs**

1. The amount of radiation absorbed per gram of tissue is referred to as a:
- a. rad.
- b. rem.
- c. mrem.
- d. Roentgen.

2. When referring to imaging in dentistry, what does CBCT stand for?
- a. Central-beam classification technology
- b. Cone-beam computed tomography
- c. Center-balanced computer technology
- d. Coronal-beam central topography

3. When the kilovoltage or kV setting in the tubehead is increased:
- a. Electrons move from the anode to the cathode with more speed.
- b. X-rays move from the anode to the cathode with more speed.
- c. Electrons move from the cathode to the anode with more speed.
- d. X-rays move from the cathode to the anode with more speed.

4. When exposing dental images in a dental operatory, what is the purpose of using barriers and disinfecting the treatment room following each patient?
- a. To reduce the susceptibility of the dental patient's immune system in order to lessen disease transmission potential
- b. To limit the types of portals or openings that exist for a pathogen to enter the dental patient and cause an infectious disease
- c. To improve time management for the dental team by allowing for shorter dental operatory turnover times between patients
- d. To eliminate or reduce the number of pathogens that are present due to aerosols of oral and respiratory fluids produced during dental imaging

5. Which of the following are correct in regard to the different wavelengths produced in dentistry?
- a. X-rays with longer wavelength have less penetrating power.
- b. X-rays with shorter wavelength have less penetrating power.
- c. X-rays with shorter wavelengths are more likely to be absorbed by matter prior to striking the image receptor.
- d. X-rays with longer wavelengths can be referred to as hard rays.

6. Using the proper _____ assists in controlling the amount of radiation emitted to the patient.

    a. exposure factors
    b. size film
    c. monitoring device
    d. time management

7. Which of the following types of radiation is also known as "useful radiation?"

    a. Secondary radiation.
    b. Primary radiation.
    c. Tertiary radiation.
    d. Scattered radiation.

8. According to the National Council on Radiation Protection and Measurements, what is the maximum permissible dose of radiation that a dental auxiliary can receive in 1 year?

    a. 4 rems.
    b. 5 rems.
    c. 6 rems.
    d. 7 rems.

9. A cone-shaped radiopaque image on a panoramic x-ray is likely caused by:

    a. Use of a thyroid collar during imaging
    b. Earrings
    c. Orthodontic retainer
    d. Tongue piercing

10. Which one of the following is an advantage of the paralleling technique?

    a. Receptor placement is simple and easy to duplicate.
    b. Patient discomfort is minimal during dental imaging.
    c. The paralleling technique can be done without the use of any receptor placement tool, thereby reducing infection control requirements.
    d. The paralleling technique is easy to use with patients who have a low roof of the mouth or bony growths in the mouth.

11. When exposing periapical images on a young child, what size image receptor should the dental auxiliary choose?

    a. Size 0.
    b. Size 1.
    c. Size 2.
    d. Size 3.

12. What is the correct way for a dental assistant to wear a dosimeter?

    a. Only when he/she is taking x-rays
    b. All day, every day
    c. Just during normal business hours for the practice
    d. Only when he/she is at the dental office

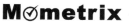

13. Which of the following images needs to show the entire tooth from 2-3 mm beyond the apex to the entire occlusal or incisal edge?

    a. Occlusal image.

    b. Bitewing image.

    c. Periapical image.

    d. Panoramic image.

14. Which of the following is not an effective way that the "as low as reasonably achievable" (ALARA) principle can be achieved in the dental office for the protection of the patient?

    a. Use of lead aprons and thyroid collars

    b. Use of D film

    c. Minimize the time of exposure

    d. Use of digital radiographs

15. When the bisecting technique is used, which of the following angles is bisected?

    a. The angle formed by the image receptor and the long axis of the tooth.

    b. The angle formed by the central ray and the tooth

    c. The angle formed by the central ray and the image receptor.

    d. The angle that is perpendicular to the image receptor.

16. Which of the following is a direct result when an image receptor is exposed with a high milliamperage or mA setting?

    a. High contrast.

    b. Low contrast.

    c. High density.

    d. Low density.

17. When classifying patient care items based on their potential to spread infection due to their intended use, which classification is the Snap-A-Ray?

    a. Critical instrument

    b. Semicritical instrument

    c. Noncritical instrument

    d. Due to its use in dental imaging and the minimal risk of it transmitting disease, it is not classified into one of these classifications.

18. Determine which of the following statements is TRUE:

    a. Patients must have a complete series of x-rays taken once a year.

    b. Dental images should not be taken on a "routine basis."

    c. Multiple attempts at obtaining a diagnostically acceptable radiograph should be made until an attempt is successful.

    d. Informed consent is not needed for exposing routine dental x-rays.

19. During production of dental x-rays inside the dental tube, which component is responsible for creating thermionic emission?

    a. The tungsten target.

    b. The filament circuit.

    c. The step-up transformer.

    d. The anode.

DANB Practice Test

20. Which of the following is correct regarding a radiation monitoring badge?

    a. It is a device that can measure the amount of radiation that reaches the body of the radiographer.

    b. It consists of calcium tungstate crystals that are sensitive to secondary radiation.

    c. It is worn by the dental assistant for a minimum of 4 months and then sent in for processing.

    d. The badge should be stored in the dental operatory where the radiation exposures take place.

21. When the bisecting technique is used, foreshortening will occur if the central ray is directed perpendicular to the:

    a. plane of the image receptor.

    b. imaginary bisector.

    c. long axis of the tooth on the same arch.

    d. long axis of the tooth in the opposite arch.

22. Which of the following images has the purpose of demonstrating the buccal-lingual and anterior-posterior relationships of structures on an image receptor?

    a. Lateral cephalometric image.

    b. Occlusal image.

    c. Periapical image.

    d. Waters projection.

23. During extraoral panoramic dental radiography, if the chin is positioned too high or tipped inward:

    a. the Curve of Spee will be correctly aligned.

    b. the Frankfort plane is positioned too high.

    c. the Frankfort plane is positioned too low and is tipped in a downward direction.

    d. the final processed panoramic will have increased definition in the area of the maxillary teeth.

24. Which of the following best describes cone beam computed tomography (CBCT)?

    a. The smallest element of three-dimensional imaging, also known as a volume element pixel.

    b. A term used to describe computer-assisted digital imaging in dentistry.

    c. A technique that uses a cone-shaped x-ray beam to gather information and present it in three dimensions on a computer screen.

    d. The reconstruction of raw data into images when imported into a specific viewing software.

25. Which of the following choices is NOT a type of somatic cell?

    a. Brain cells.

    b. Kidney cells.

    c. Reproductive cells.

    d. Liver cells.

26. Indicate which of the following statements is TRUE:

    a. All dental x-rays pass through the patient's skin and reach the dental film.

    b. The skin tissues of the patient being radiographed absorb all x-rays.

    c. The skin tissues of the patient being radiographed absorb some x-rays.

    d. No dental x-rays pass through the patient's skin and reach the dental film.

27. A patient is being prepared for a panoramic exposure. The patient is wearing an earring in the left ear only. The exposure is made and the panoramic radiograph is processed. Where will the earring artifact be seen on the panoramic film?

a. The earring will be seen on the right side of the film, slightly higher than the real object.
b. The earring will be seen on the left side of the film, slightly higher than the real object.
c. The earring will be seen in the area of the anterior mandibular teeth.
d. The earring will be seen on the right side of the film, slightly lower than the real object.

28. Which type of x-rays is removed by the aluminum disks found within the x-ray tube head?

a. Low energy, short wavelength.
b. Low energy, long wavelength.
c. High energy, long wavelength.
d. High energy, short wavelength.

29. Under state laws, the *respondeat superior* doctrine states that:

a. the employee is responsible for his or her own actions when taking a dental radiograph.
b. the employer is responsible for the actions of the radiographer when taking a dental radiograph.
c. the patient is responsible for the actions of the dental radiographer.
d. the state is responsible for the actions of the dental radiographer.

30. Which of the following is worn by the dental auxiliary in order to measure radiation exposure?

a. Particulate monitor.
b. Dosimeter.
c. Radiation shield.
d. Ionization badge.

31. When considering hand hygiene practices that may be used during dental imaging, which one of the following is the most accurate?

a. A routine hand washing should include using water and nonantimicrobial soap, washing the hands for 20–30 seconds followed by a long rinse with water from the fingertips to the wrists.
b. An alcohol-based hand rub should be used and rubbed between the hands and fingers, covering all areas until the hands are completely dry.
c. A soap product should be selected that has antimicrobial properties and is used with water for 10 seconds of hand washing.
d. A routine hand wash should be performed for 20–30 seconds followed by an alcohol-based hand rub until the hands are completely dry.

32. Determine which of the following statements is TRUE regarding the standard of care that is provided by a dentist:

a. Documentation signed by the patient, releasing the dental provider from liability, protects the dentist when treating a patient who refuses dental x-rays.
b. Dentists are allowed to treat a patient even though the patient refuses necessary dental x-rays.
c. Legally, a patient cannot consent to negligent care.
d. Legally, a patient can consent to negligent care.

DANB Practice Test

33. How far does the dental auxiliary need to stand from the source of radiation in order to prevent exposure to secondary radiation?

    a. 3 feet.
    b. 4 feet.
    c. 5 feet.
    d. 6 feet.

34. Characteristics of x-rays include all of the following EXCEPT:

    a. X-rays are not visible or apparent to any of the senses
    b. X-rays travel at half the speed of light
    c. X-rays travel in a straight line but can easily be deflected
    d. Shorter x-rays are more useful in dental radiographs

35. Which one of the following is the name of the infection precaution measure used in dentistry to ensure that all patients are treated in the same manner for infection control practices?

    a. Standard precautions
    b. Universal precautions
    c. Medical precautions
    d. Contact precautions

36. When capturing dental images, which one of the following is an example of how infectious diseases can be spread directly from patient to patient?

    a. Using a contaminated XCP device for sensor placement
    b. Glove puncture in the dental assistant's gloves during placement of the sensor
    c. The dental assistant wearing a mask below the nose when capturing images
    d. Failing to have the patient wear protective eyewear during image exposure

37. Which one of the following statements describes the correct infection control guidelines to follow when capturing dental images with a wired sensor?

    a. After using the wired sensor to capture digital images, the first step in processing the sensor is to place it in the ultrasonic machine for a minimum of 10 minutes.
    b. The wired sensors do not require the use of a barrier because they can be sterilized with the autoclave and/or chemiclave.
    c. When using a wired sensor during digital imaging, a barrier covering the sensor and the wired connection is required along with disinfection of the wired sensor after use.
    d. Avoid the use of a plastic finger cot when using wired sensors due to the compression that the finger cot places on the sensor.

38. When taking which of the following images does the dental radiographer need to ensure that the interproximal areas and the bone levels are adequately captured and demonstrated along with the coronal surfaces of the teeth?

    a. Reverse Towne image.
    b. Posteroanterior image.
    c. Bitewing image.
    d. Periapical image.

39. Which one of the following best describes the purpose of the panoramic digital image?

a. To look at the length of the back teeth
b. To look at the upper and lower jaws and teeth
c. To view the inner areas of the ear
d. To look for dental decay

40. All of the following apply to the lead apron EXCEPT:

a. It is recommended for both intraoral and extraoral image receptors.
b. It is intended to protect the reproductive and blood-forming organs.
c. It is a device that prevents radiation from reaching radiosensitive organs.
d. It was developed with the main purpose of shielding the patient from leakage and stray radiation.

41. Which one of the following agencies developed and released the 2003 Guidelines for Infection Control in Dental Health-Care Settings that apply to dental radiography and include paid and unpaid dental professionals?

a. Occupational Safety and Health Administration (OSHA)
b. Centers for Disease Control and Prevention (CDC)
c. Organization for Safety, Asepsis, and Prevention (OSAP)
d. American Dental Association (ADA)

42. A dental assistant is seeing a patient who is having pain in a front tooth. The patient states that it is a throbbing and aching pain that prevents sleep at night. Which one of the following techniques is most effective at capturing all of the areas that the dentist will need to view in the correct dimensions?

a. Bisecting
b. Occlusal
c. Bitewing
d. Paralleling

43. When using the bisecting technique, which one of the following is correct?

a. The digital receptor is placed on the facial surface of the tooth to allow for optimal patient comfort.
b. The digital receptor must be placed parallel to the tooth.
c. The dental assistant must visualize and use an imaginary angle.
d. The dental assistant must use a bisecting digital system when performing this technique.

44. Which one of the following is considered the most important infection control law in dentistry and exists to protect employees from occupational exposure to blood and other potentially infectious materials?

a. Morbidity and Mortality Weekly Report infection control guidelines
b. Hazard Communication Standard
c. Employee Right-to-Know Law
d. Bloodborne Pathogens Standard

45. **Which of the following is considered secondary radiation?**
    a. Radiation that goes through the collimator and position-indicating device (PID)
    b. Radiation that reflects off the patient's face
    c. Radiation that leaks from the tubehead
    d. Radiation directed at an area for cancer treatment

46. **If the milliamp (mA) setting is increased on the dental radiograph x-ray control panel, what will the overall effect be on the density of the processed dental film?**
    a. The processed dental film will have decreased density.
    b. The processed dental film will have increased density.
    c. The processed dental film will have decreased contrast.
    d. The processed dental film will have increased contrast.

47. **When positioning the patient for panoramic exposure, the Frankfort plane should be positioned:**
    a. perpendicular to the floor.
    b. parallel to the floor.
    c. perpendicular to the cassette.
    d. parallel to the cassette.

48. **Which of the following structures will appear as a radiolucent area on a dental radiograph?**
    a. Coronoid process.
    b. Incisive foramen.
    c. Genial tubercles.
    d. Zygomatic process.

49. **When considering personal protective equipment (PPE) and dental imaging, which one of the following practices must be followed to limit the risk of disease transmission?**
    a. When spatter and aerosols are likely, the dental assistant must wear a surgical mask and protective eyewear or a chin-length face shield.
    b. It is not required to wash face shields and dental eyewear after dental imaging or patient treatment because these PPE items are not directly touched and have no ability to spread infection.
    c. An N95 respirator face mask should be worn for all dental imaging procedures due to the proximity of the dental assistant to the patient's oral cavity.
    d. Protective clothing is not required for the process of capturing dental images because minimal spatter is generated.

50. **What type of radiograph is used by an orthodontist to assist with treatment planning?**
    a. Tomography
    b. Sialography
    c. Cephalometric
    d. Occlusal

51. Which of the following can be defined as tiny particles of matter that possess mass and travel in straight lines and at high speeds?

- a. Electromagnetic radiation.
- b. Radioactive radiation matter.
- c. Particulate radiation.
- d. X-radiation.

52. Short teeth with blunted roots appear on the image receptor when:

- a. the horizontal angulation is incorrect.
- b. the occlusal plane is misaligned.
- c. there is collimator cutoff.
- d. the vertical angulation is excessive.

53. The best radiograph to obtain for diagnosis of temporomandibular joint (TMJ) is:

- a. Panoramic
- b. Periapical
- c. Sialography
- d. Arthrography

54. Which of the following is controlled by the milliamperage or mA setting found on the control panel of a dental tubehead?

- a. The speed of the x-rays that hit the image receptor.
- b. The size of the x-rays that hit the image receptor.
- c. The shape of the x-rays that hit the image receptor.
- d. The number of x-rays that hit the image receptor.

55. A critical organ(s) affected by cumulative radiation exposure is/are:

- a. the mucosa of the mouth.
- b. the bones of the hand.
- c. the lens of the eye.
- d. the nostrils.

56. When using the paralleling technique during periapical exposure:

- a. the central ray of the beam is perpendicular to the tooth and film.
- b. the central ray of the beam is parallel to the long axis of the tooth and film.
- c. the central ray of the beam is at a 45-degree angle to the tooth and film.
- d. the central ray of the beam is at a 65-degree angle to the tooth and film.

57. During a patient exam, the dentist requests that the dental assistant capture an image that will show the complete apices and the full crowns of teeth #8 and #9 to evaluate pain that the patient is experiencing. Which dental image should the dental assistant capture?

- a. Occlusal
- b. Bitewing
- c. Periapical
- d. Panoramic

58. A bitewing radiograph is LEAST useful in diagnosing:

   a. An impacted tooth
   b. Tooth decay
   c. Periodontal bone loss
   d. Gum disease

59. All of the following are part of the panoramic head positioning device EXCEPT:

   a. notched bite block.
   b. forehead rest.
   c. lateral head guides.
   d. the cassette.

60. Which one of the following is correct regarding the object-receptor distance in dental imaging?

   a. The object-receptor distance is the space between the tooth and the imaging sensor used by the dental staff.
   b. The receptor should be placed outside the lip, which determines the appropriate object-receptor distance.
   c. When using this distance as a guide in digital imaging, it is referred to as the long-cone technique.
   d. The object-receptor distance is only considered when taking panoramic images.

61. What is NOT an advantage of the paralleling technique?

   a. Structures on the image will have sharp detail.
   b. Minimal enlargement of teeth structures.
   c. Images will have increased clarity and contrast.
   d. Comfortable for the patient and easy to place the image receptor for operator.

62. When considering the use of surface barriers in the treatment room during dental imaging, which one of the following is correct?

   a. Surface barriers are required for use in dentistry and must be present in every patient treatment to prevent the spread of aerosolized pathogens.
   b. Smooth, hard surfaces including countertops, dental imaging trays, light handles and supply containers should always be covered with barriers due to their proximity to patient care.
   c. The electrical switches of the imaging exposure button and the dental tubehead should be covered with barriers, when possible, to prevent contamination.
   d. When surface barriers are used and remain intact during a procedure, the dental assistant must disinfect all areas under the barriers after the procedure is complete.

63. Which federal law requires that all persons who operate x-ray machinery to produce dental radiographs are properly trained and certified?

   a. OSHA.
   b. JADA.
   c. FDA.
   d. The Consumer-Patient Radiation Health and Safety Act.

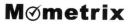

64. Which of the following statements is TRUE regarding the use of cotton rolls and image receptor holding devices during the placement of the image receptor and radiation exposure?

    a. Plastic image receptor holding devices are not advised during radiation exposure due to the radiopaque distortion they create on the resulting image.

    b. Cotton roll holders should be used in all cases where cotton rolls are placed in the mouth in order to prevent shifting during radiation exposure.

    c. Cotton roll can be placed in an edentulous area to aid in stabilizing the image receptor during exposure.

    d. Styrofoam image receptor holding devices are outdated and should no longer be used during radiation exposure.

65. Which one of the following is an effective method of sterilizing patient care items used in dental imaging, uses water steam under pressure, prevents corrosion, and produces dry patient care items once the cycle is complete?

    a. Unsaturated chemical vapor

    b. Static air sterilizer

    c. Forced air sterilizer

    d. Steam autoclave

66. Who of the following would be the most sensitive to the effects of radiation?

    a. 2-year-old child.

    b. 15-year-old teenager.

    c. 25-year-old man.

    d. Developing fetus.

67. An XCP device is an example of what type of control used in dentistry that can be described as equipment or a device used to minimize employee exposure?

    a. Work practice control

    b. Engineering control

    c. Administrative control

    d. Sensor placement control

68. What is the function of the collimator?

    a. It directs the x-ray beam to the appropriate place

    b. It allows the electrons to cross over the cathode to reach the anode

    c. It forms the shape and size of the x-ray beam upon leaving the tubehead

    d. It filters out the wavelengths that are unusable

69. The American Academy of Oral and Maxillofacial Radiology recommends using the _____ technique, which will provide the dentist with the most accurate image with the least amount of distortion.

    a. bitewing

    b. paralleling

    c. bisecting angle

    d. extraoral

DANB Practice Test

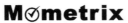

70. When identifying anatomical structures and dental materials on radiograph, which of the following is TRUE?

    a. The enamel is radiolucent and located at the crown of the tooth
    b. The root canals are radiopaque and extend from the pulp chamber to the apex of the tooth
    c. The periodontal ligament can be visualized as radiopaque
    d. The dentin is not as radiopaque as enamel

71. Which one of the following best defines microorganisms that can be spread during dental imaging and are capable of causing disease?

    a. Bacteria
    b. Pathogens
    c. Protozoa
    d. Biofilms

72. Legally, dental images, as part of the patient's dental record, are the property of:

    a. the patient.
    b. the patient's caretaker.
    c. the dentist.
    d. the insurance company.

73. Which of the following structures would appear radiopaque on a processed dental periapical x-ray?

    a. The orbit of the eye
    b. The nasal septum
    c. The mucosa of the cheek
    d. Dentin

74. When processing an XCP device after patient use, which one of the following is an acceptable method of precleaning that works by using high-frequency sound waves to loosen and remove debris?

    a. Holding solution
    b. Ultrasonic cleaning
    c. Hand scrubbing
    d. Instrument washing machine

75. Under what circumstances may the dental auxiliary hold a digital receptor in a patient's mouth during exposure?

    a. The dental auxiliary should never hold an image receptor in a patient's mouth during exposure.
    b. When the child is a minor and the parent is not present.
    c. When the patient is physically handicapped and is unable to keep the image receptor in their mouth.
    d. During emergency surgeries when the patient is unconscious.

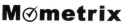

76. What is the lowest level disinfectant that can be used for the disinfection of clinical contact surfaces, including the dental tubehead and dental operatory where images are captured?

    a. Sterilant level
    b. High level
    c. Intermediate level
    d. Low level

77. When mounting processed radiographs, which anatomical landmark can assist you in mounting the mandibular premolar periapical?

    a. The mental foramen.
    b. The genial tubercles.
    c. The lingual foramen.
    d. The maxillary sinus.

78. Disproportionate changes in the size of an image on a processed radiograph are caused by:

    a. improper placement of the film prior to exposure.
    b. too large of a film size having been used.
    c. excessive or insufficient horizontal angulation.
    d. excessive or insufficient vertical angulation.

79. Which of the following is used to control the degree of penetration of the x-ray beam?

    a. Exposure button
    b. Kilovoltage peak selector
    c. Milliamperage selector
    d. Master switch

80. Which of the following projections are used to evaluate facial growth and development, trauma, and disease, and developmental abnormalities that may occur in the cranium?

    a. Waters projection.
    b. Submentovertex projection.
    c. Transcranial projection.
    d. Lateral cephalometric projection.

Answer Key and Explanations

1. A: A rad stands for radiation absorbed dose and can be defined as the amount of radiation that is absorbed by the tissue following an exposure. Rem stands for roentgen equivalent man, and measures the biological effect radiation may have on a patient. A roentgen measures the quantity of radiation that produces an electrical charge in the air.

2. B: CBCT stands for cone-beam computed tomography. This type of imaging is now common in dentistry for viewing parts of the face and mouth that was not possible in the past. It involves the use of various equipment ranging from a machine to take the picture, a computer to view the images, and a keyboard and software to edit and send the images to specialty providers when needed.

3. C: The kilovolt setting in the dental tubehead controls how fast the electrons and resulting x-rays travel. When this setting is increased, the electrons move from the negative side of the tubehead, the cathode side, to the positive side of the tubehead, the anode, at a greater speed and therefore exit the tubehead at a greater speed. This causes the resulting image to have a lower contrast as the x-rays are able to penetrate more objects in the oral cavity.

4. D: The use of barriers when disinfecting treatment rooms following each patient is a required step in infection control in each dental office. When barriers are properly used and maintained during image exposure, they prevent microbes and pathogens from reaching the dental equipment that they are covering, eliminating the risk of disease transmission. In areas where barriers are not used, or if barriers are compromised during dental treatment, the added process of properly disinfecting each treatment room is required in order to reduce the number of pathogens present on the dental equipment before the next patient can be seen. Time management should not be considered in the implementation of infection control practices because patient safety comes first. Barrier use and the use of disinfectants do not reduce the susceptibility of a patient's immune system nor do they limit the types of portals or openings that exist for microbes to enter a patient.

5. A: Different types of x-rays can be produced by the dental tubehead. X-rays with longer wavelengths have less penetrating power due to the longer wavelengths, and are commonly referred to as soft waves. X-rays with shorter wavelengths that are moving faster and therefore have greater penetrating power are known as hard waves due to how they interact with the objects they strike.

6. A: Using the proper exposure factors assists in controlling the amount of radiation emitted to the patient. The monitoring device is a tool used to measure the possibility of radiation exposure to the employee. Time management is a useful tool to accomplish tasks with efficiency and quality.

7. B: Primary radiation is known as "useful radiation," which produces the latent image needed. All other radiation that is produced by the exposure is not beneficial to the radiograph, the radiographer, or the patient. Much of this non-beneficial radiation is filtered out by the aluminum disks even before the primary bean is emitted from the PID.

8. B: The dental auxiliary, or anyone who may be occupationally exposed to radiation, has a maximum amount of radiation that they should be exposed to. The National Council on Radiation Protection and Measurements has deemed that a dental auxiliary should not be exposed to more than 5 rem in a 1-year time period. Anything beyond this increases the chances that biological damage may occur, and has been labeled as unsafe.

104

9. A: Incorrect placement of a lead apron or thyroid collar use during panoramic x-rays will likely cause a radiopaque image of a cone that will likely block the mandible. A lead apron without a thyroid collar should always be used for proper imaging. Ghost images seen on the panoramic radiograph can be caused by earrings, glasses, removable dentures, or retainers. Hearing aids and any other type of metallic objects can also cause a ghost image. A ghost image is a whitish looking image of the item that appears on the opposite side of the film. The image usually appears blurry and is larger than the actual item. Any of the aforementioned items should be removed, if possible, prior to the panoramic x-ray being taken.

10. A: The paralleling technique is one that is easy for the dental radiographer to do again and again. It does not involve complex rules and angles and simply involves placing the digital sensor next to the tooth on the inside of the mouth so the two are in the same plane. Other techniques require the use of stricter procedures and protocols that must be practiced before they can be implemented.

11. A: When the dental auxiliary is exposing radiographs on a young child, both periapical or bitewing images, a size 0 imaging receptor should be used due to how small a young child's mouth may be. If a larger size is used, the child may be unable to close properly, causing possible distortion to the image.

12. D: A dosimeter is a radiation monitoring device that is used to measure occupational exposure to radiation. The most common types are film badges or pocket dosimeters. A dental assistant will most likely be assigned a dosimeter to wear. The correct procedure is to wear the device only when at the dental office. It should be removed when leaving the building because sunshine can alter the results. The purpose of the device is to measure occupational exposure, not all radiation exposure during everyday living. The device is turned into the monitoring company at the end of the reporting period, which is typically about 3-4 weeks. The company keeps track of the accumulated radiation exposure for employees quarterly, annually, and over the course of their lifetimes.

13. C: When the dentist needs to view the entire occlusal or incisal edge as well as the apex of a tooth, they will request that a periapical image be taken on the patient. This image requires that, along with the required structures or teeth, that the entire tooth is shown, including the occlusal or incisal edge as well as 2-3 mm beyond the apex in order to determine if there is any periapical lesion in that area.

14. B: Dental radiographs are important but they are a source of radiation exposure to the patient and should be used appropriately. A 2-4 bitewing x-ray will provide about 0.005 mSv. This is not much considering that the average person may be exposed to 3.2 mSv over the course of a year from everyday sources. The ALARA ("as low as reasonably achievable") principle should be followed in dental offices. This incorporates trying to minimize the amount of radiation exposure within the dental office. For patients, the use of lead apron and thyroid collar helps to cut down on exposure. Using an F film speed also helps because this is the fastest speed and it reduces exposure by up to 60%. A reduction in the size of the x-ray beam is important for reducing radiation exposure. The beam should only be as large as the image receptor. Proper processing procedures are also important.

15. A: When the bisecting technique is used, the dental auxiliary must determine what angle they are going to use to aim their central ray at during exposure. This angle is determined by bisecting or dividing in half the angle formed by the long axis of the tooth and the image receptor. This angle is called the imaginary bisecting angle because it does not physically exist, but is created by the dental auxiliary. When the central ray is aimed at this imaginary bisector angle, the end result will be an image receptor with adequate diagnostic capabilities.

16. C: When a high milliamperage (mA) setting is used, the direct effect is an image that will demonstrate high density. This is due to more electrons being created at the tungsten filament, which directly results in more x-rays being created. When there are more x-rays, more are allowed to strike the image receptor and the image will be darker.

17. B: Snap-A-Rays are sensor-holding devices used in dental imaging and are classified as semicritical instruments. These devices hold a digital sensor during placement into the oral cavity during dental imaging. They touch the mucous membranes of the oral tissue but do not penetrate soft tissue or bone; therefore, they have a lower risk for disease transmission. Most brands of sensor holders are heat tolerant—as semicritical instruments, they should be sterilized by heat. Other examples of semicritical instruments used in dental imaging include the XCP device and other reusable receptor-holding items.

18. B: The only true statement is as follows: "Dental images should not be taken on a 'routine basis.'" The rationale for this statement being true is that dental radiographic imaging should only be used as a tool of diagnosis when pathology is considered. To further explain this statement, we must remember that as healthcare professionals, we are to follow the "as low as reasonably achievable" (ALARA) concept. Radiographic images should not be taken on a routine basis as indicated by an insurance policy or as a means of generating office revenue. Images should be taken only when a defined measure is needed to maintain the health of the patient.

19. B: During production of the dental x-rays inside the dental tube, the cathode filament circuit is responsible for creating thermionic emission. The step-up transformer is directly associated with the source of electrical flow into the dental tube. This energy created by the electrical circuit from the wall outlet immediately charges the cathode filament circuit, making charged electrons available to be emitted as x-rays through the position-indicating device (PID).

20. A: A radiation monitoring badge, commonly referred to as a dosimeter, is a device that is worn at waist level by a dental auxiliary during their time at the dental office. This device measures the amount of radiation that they are exposed to. It contains a piece of film inside of a plastic case that is sensitive to radiation. After a specified amount of time, this device is sent in for analysis and a report is generated and sent back to the dental auxiliary describing the results.

21. A: When using the bisecting technique, the dental auxiliary needs to aim the central ray at the imaginary bisecting line that is created by the long axis of the tooth and the plane of the image receptor. If the central ray is instead aimed at the plane of the image receptor itself, the resulting image will have foreshortening and may need to be retaken in order to reduce the vertical angulations used.

22. B: The occlusal image is taken when the dentist needs to view structures using the third dimension or needs to see things using the buccal-lingual relationships. This image allows the dentist to determine depth when looking at structures, compared with periapical images, which do not allow for adequate depth perception of oral structures.

23. B: During extraoral panoramic dental radiography, if the chin is positioned too high or tipped inward, the Frankfort plane is too high. With this improper positioning of the chin, a reverse smile line may be seen on the processed radiograph. The patient should be positioned so that the Frankfort plane is parallel to the floor to avoid numerous negative effects that may result on the processed radiograph.

24. C: Cone beam computer tomography (CBCT) is a technique that is increasing in popularity in the medical and dental fields. This type of imaging works by using a cone-shaped x-ray beam to expose a patient. This information is then gathered and interpreted by a computer system, resulting in an image that is presented in three dimensions on a computer screen.

25. C: Somatic cells are all cells found in the body except the reproductive cells. The female ova and the male sperm are examples of the reproductive cells, with brain cells, kidney cells, and liver cells being examples of somatic cells.

26. C: The following statement is the only statement that is TRUE: The skin tissues of the patient being radiographed absorb some x-rays. Not all of the x-rays completed come in contact with the patient. Scattered x-rays may immediately diverge from the position-indicating device (PID) and never reach the patient. But those x-rays that are directed at the patient do come in contact with the patient's skin.

27. A: The earring, worn in the left ear, will appear as an artifact in the right side of the film, and it will be slightly higher than the real object. This image is often known as a ghost image.

28. B: Low-energy, long-wavelength x-rays are removed by the aluminum disks found within the x-ray tube head. These long, low-energy wavelengths provide no benefit to the x-ray beam that exits the tube head via the position-indicating device (PID).

29. B: Under state laws, the *respondeat superior* doctrine states that the employer is responsible for the actions of the dental radiographer. Ultimately, the employer is responsible for a person working in his or her office under his or her direction. An employee has the responsibility of following the directions of the employer and must understand that his or her work in taking radiographs is basically an extension of the provider's work. Providers will hold the dental staff responsible for their work, but ultimately, if there is a legal situation pertaining to the care of a patient, it is the employer that would be responsible. It must be noted that this varies from state to state because many states require dental radiographers to be licensed.

30. B: A radiation monitoring badge, commonly referred to as a dosimeter, is a device that is worn by the dental auxiliary during the traditional workday at a dental clinic. This is a device that measures any amounts of radiation that the dental auxiliary may be exposed to. This is something that should not be worn outside of the dental office as it may capture other sources of radiation and distort the final amounts. After the specified time period, a week, a month, or a quarter, this device is then sent in for a final analysis, and the results are then sent to the dental auxiliary for interpretation.

31. B: Hand hygiene is the most important component of minimizing disease transmission from patient to patient. Using an alcohol-based hand rub and rubbing it into the hands until they are completely dry is required before donning and after doffing gloves for dental imaging. It is the rubbing motion that helps make the product effective; it is important to continue the rubbing action until the hands are dry. When the skin has come in contact with bodily fluid such as that in the oral cavity, a hand wash with soap is required. A routine hand wash with nonantimicrobial soap is acceptable, but the length of time for that hand wash must be 40–60 seconds. The use of antimicrobial soaps and products is acceptable for a minimal of 15 seconds in order to be effective.

32. C: Regarding the standard of care that is provided by a dentist, a patient cannot consent to negligent care. The statement, "Documentation signed by the patient, releasing the dental provider from liability, protects the dentist when treating a patient who refuses dental x-rays," is a false statement because the dentist providing treatment will/can be liable for any negligence should a

107

procedure result in a negative outcome. The statement "Dentists are allowed to treat a patient even though the patient refuses necessary dental x-rays" is also false because an ethical practicing dentist will not attempt to treat a patient who refuses dental x-rays because dental x-rays are a vital tool in the proper diagnosis and treatment of every patient.

33. D: In order to prevent any secondary or scatter radiation from striking the dental auxiliary, they should stand at least 6 feet away from the source of radiation or the tubehead during any type of radiation exposure, both intraoral and extraoral.

34. B: X-rays are a type of energy that are able to penetrate matter. They are classified as electromagnetic radiation. Other types of electromagnetic radiation include television waves, radio, radar, and light. Shorter x-rays are more useful in dental radiographs because the penetrate structures more easily than longer wavelengths. X-rays travel at the speed of light. They are not detectable by any of the senses. X-rays do not contain mass or weight and do not contain a charge. X-rays travel in a straight line but are easily deflected to other areas. X-rays are either absorbed by matter or scattered and can cause damage due to secondary radiation exposure.

35. A: Standard precautions refer to the general infection prevention measures that should be used with all patients in dentistry and in medicine. Using standard precautions ensures that even in relatively low infection risk patients, standardized measures are used to protect the patient and dental team from disease transmission. These include the proper use of hand hygiene and personal protective equipment (PPE).

36. A: When capturing dental images, it is essential that the dental team use properly sterilized instruments and receptor holders. The extension cone paralleling (XCP) device (often referred to as a Rinn device, after one manufacturer) is a common dental instrument that is used to position a digital sensor in the patient's oral cavity when capturing dental images. This item must be properly precleaned and heat sterilized between patients. If this does not happen, or if the sterilization process is ineffective or done incorrectly, it will render the dental item unsterile. This can directly cause the spread of infectious diseases from one patient to another because the pathogens may still be on the item when it is used on the next patient. If the dental assistant has a glove puncture or is improperly wearing their personal protective equipment (PPE), this can lead to disease transmission from the dental assistant to the patient or from the patient to the dental assistant. Eye protection is not required nor does it serve any purpose for the patient during image production.

37. C: Wired sensors cannot be placed into an autoclave, chemiclave, or dry heat; they should be processed by other forms of submersion, heat, or pressure sterilization methods. When used, wired sensors must be covered completely with a barrier that extends past the area where the sensor and the wire connect. After use, the barrier should be removed and the sensor needs to be disinfected according to the manufacturer's directions. Wired sensors cannot be placed in the ultrasonic machine because they are electronic devices and will be damaged. Plastic barriers can tear or leak after a few exposures; therefore, finger cots are recommended to provide extra support and will not compromise the wired sensor.

38. C: Bitewing images are the images of choice when the dentist needs to view the interproximal areas of the teeth or when the dentist or dental hygienist needs to view the bone levels in the mouth. When taken with correct vertical and horizontal angulations, these images provide the most accurate view of these structures.

39. B: The panoramic dental digital picture is one that will show the upper and lower portions of the mouth in one image. Not only will bone be in the picture, it will also include parts of the jaw and the eye sockets; the dental radiographer may even see parts of the spine.

40. D: Lead aprons may be required for use in some states and optional in others. Regardless of the requirement to wear a lead apron, they can be worn for both intraoral and extraoral images. They are intended to protect the reproductive and blood-producing cells in the body and to prevent radiation from reaching radiosensitive organs. They are also used to prevent primary and secondary radiation from striking the patients.

41. B: The CDC created the 2003 Guidelines for Infection Control in Dental Health-Care Settings in collaboration with other agencies involved with patient and worker safety. Although these guidelines are from 2003, they are still applicable and referenced today. They contain recommendations that apply to dentistry that are upheld by state boards and authoritative agencies and serve as the best practices for dental care. OSHA is a regulatory agency that serves to protect workers in the United States. The ADA is a national agency composed of dentists across the United States. OSAP is an agency composed of dental professionals, researchers, consultants, and other staff who serve with the goal of providing evidence-based practices on infection control and safety.

42. D: The dental assistant should always use the paralleling technique when needing to view the entire tooth. This is the technique that will show the tooth in the most realistic dimensions possible when viewing a single tooth This will allow the dentist to have a realistic picture to view the dental anatomy and develop a treatment plan that is best for the patient and will provide the most relief for his or her discomfort.

43. C: When using the bisecting technique, the dental assistant will use angles that must be visualized as abstract angles versus the angles that are created when placing the sensor in the mouth. This is because, when using this technique, the mouth is preventing the sensor from being placed at a right angle, which is needed to produce images that are dimensionally accurate.

44. D: The OSHA Bloodborne Pathogens Standard is used to help protect employees from exposure to microbes that can lead to disease. Employers have a duty to provide a safe working environment for staff and are required to implement safety practices that are listed in this standard. The OSHA Hazard Communication Standard, also known as the Employee Right-to-Know Law, is another important standard that protects employees from hazardous chemicals. The CDC's Morbidity and Mortality Weekly Report infection control guidelines have been developed as recommendations for safety in dentistry and are best practices.

45. B: A dental assistant can be exposed to 3 types of radiation. Primary radiation can be received directly from the x-ray machine; the beam that originates from the x-ray tube and goes through the collimator and position-indicating device (PID) is used for obtaining dental radiographs. Secondary radiation is that received because of scatter radiation, which is deflected away. This can occur when radiation hits the patient's face and bounces off. Leakage radiation is received if the tubehead seal is not properly secured. The goal for any dental employee is zero radiation exposure, which can be attainable if proper procedures and safety guidelines are followed.

46. B: If the milliamp (mA) setting is increased on the dental radiograph x-ray control panel, the processed film will have increased density. The mA settings on the control panel are directly related to controlling the amount of density that will be seen on the resulting radiograph. Factors including exposure time, technique used, length of the PID used, and kilovolt peak (kVp) settings will also have an effect on the density of the processed film.

Answer Key and Explanations

47. B: When positioning the patient for panoramic exposure, the Frankfort plane should be parallel to the floor. If the Frankfort plane were to be positioned perpendicular to the floor, the patient's head would have to be on its side, as if the patient were lying down on his or her side. Because the cassette of the panoramic unit is constantly rotating during the exposure, the patient's Frankfort plane cannot be positioned parallel or perpendicular to the cassette because it is not a fixed object.

48. B: The incisive foramen will appear as a radiolucent area found on the maxillary central periapical image receptor. This anatomical structure appears radiolucent because a foramen is a hole or opening that allows for the passageway of nerves and vessels. The coronoid process, genial tubercles, and zygomatic process are all structures that are made from bone, and will appear radiopaque on a dental radiograph.

49. A: The dental assistant must wear a mask and eye protection or a chin-length face shield when spatter or aerosols are likely. This will provide protection from pathogens entering the eyes or the mucous membranes of the nasal cavity. The dental assistant is not required to use an N95 mask during the capturing of dental images. The Occupational Safety and Health Administration (OSHA) requires these masks to be used if treating patients who may be potentially infected with COVID-19 or other airborne diseases. These masks are available in many dental offices, but they are not required for imaging. Per OSHA guidelines, protective clothing must be worn by the dental assistant during image capturing regardless of the amount of spatter and aerosols anticipated.

50. C: An orthodontist typically uses 2 types of radiographs for treatment planning proposes. The panoramic radiograph is used to visualize the positioning of primary and permanent teeth as well as to visualize the amount of space available for emerging teeth to erupt. The cephalometric radiograph is also used. This is a type of extraoral radiograph that shows the whole side of the head including all the bones, the skull, and soft tissues. This type of x-ray allows the orthodontist to monitor for changes in the jaw as well positioning of the teeth to track treatment progress. Cephalometric radiographs are also used by otolaryngologists to visualize the airway in a patient with sleep apnea.

51. C: Particulate radiation is a type of radiation that can be defined as tiny particles of matter that do have mass or weight and travel in straight lines at high speeds. This type of radiation differs from electromagnetic radiation, which is what is produced in dentistry. Electromagnetic radiation does not possess weight or mass and cannot be seen with the naked eye.

52. D: When an image receptor is taken and appears to have short, blunted root tips, the error is foreshortening. This is caused by excessive vertical angulations and, in order to be corrected, the dental auxiliary needs to retake the image and reduce the amount of vertical angulation that were used.

53. D: The temporomandibular joint (TMJ) is located at the jaw joint. TMJ disorders can cause a range of symptoms including clicking sounds, locked jaw, headaches, and ear pain. TMJ can be quite debilitating for many patients. TMJ disorders can be caused by trauma to the TMJ, aging, grinding, or clenching of the teeth, or misalignment of the teeth that causes issues with proper bite. There is no single diagnostic test for TMJ disorders. Regular dental x-rays do not diagnose TMJ. Transcranial radiographs are sometimes used to show changes in bone structure. The patient's history of symptoms along with possible arthrography, MRI, or CAT scan may be required. Arthrography involves the use of radiographic contrast injected into the temporomandibular joint. This makes the area being visualized turn opaque to highlight the structure of the area.

54. D: The milliamperage setting (mA setting) controls the number of electrons generated by the tungsten filament, which directly controls how many x-rays will be created at the tungsten target. The mA setting does not control how fast the electrons move inside the tubehead and does not control the size or the shape of the resulting x-ray beam.

55. C: A critical organ affected by cumulative radiation exposure is the lens of the eye. Although every organ can be affected by cumulative radiation exposure, the lens of the eye is much more sensitive to this exposure than the others listed. A critical organ is one that does not have an immediate source of protection to absorb the radiation exposure. The lens of the eye does not have this protection, whereas many other organs do. The layers of skin, for example, are protective layers that must be penetrated before the radiation can reach deep internal organs.

56. A: When using the paralleling technique during periapical exposure, the central ray of the beam is perpendicular to the long axis of the tooth and film. The central ray, if positioned correctly, will be positioned at a 90-degree angle. This 90-degree angle is formed by the position-indicating device (PID) placement, perpendicular to the long axis of the tooth and the film parallel to the long axis of the tooth.

57. C: The dental assistant should expose a periapical image, which is the best choice when the dentist needs to see the entire tooth structure. The sensor is placed behind the tooth for this type of image, which will go from the tip of the tooth to the tip of the root, providing the view that the dentist will need for a correct diagnosis.

58. A: A bitewing x-ray is a type of intraoral radiograph. This type of x-ray shows the upper and lower teeth in one portion of the mouth. The range of the x-ray extends from the tooth to the crown up to the bone. It does not include the roots. Bitewing x-rays will detect tooth decay and show changes in bone density related to gum disease. Bitewings are also used to check crown placement and fillings. In order to obtain a proper bitewing radiograph, the patient must be in an upright position in the dental chair, covered with a lead apron and thyroid collar. The x-ray film is placed in the patient's mouth using a special device for film holding. The film is positioned between the upper and lower teeth of the area to be x-rayed. The patient is instructed to bite down on the film and the x-ray beam is directed towards the film. The patient should remain still during the procedure. An impacted tooth is generally diagnosed using an extraoral x-ray.

59. D: The cassette is not a part of the panoramic head-positioning device. The cassette is what is used to contain the panoramic film as it rotates around the patient during exposure. The notched bite stick, the lateral head guides, and the forehead rest are all components of the head-positioning device that help the dental assistant to correctly position the patient's head prior to exposure.

60. A: The object-receptor distance is the distance between the tooth and the sensor or receptor. Ideally, the dental radiographer should insert the sensor in a way that allows it to get as close to the tooth as possible, which will provide an image that limits the amount of size expansion or minimization of a tooth.

61. D: While the paralleling technique has many advantages, patient comfort is not one of them. In this technique, the dental auxiliary must place the image receptor parallel to the long axis of the tooth, which can create substantial patient discomfort as the image receptor may impinge upon patient tissues and oral structures.

62. C: When considering the use of surface barriers in dentistry, it is recommended to place them over hard-to-clean areas and surfaces as a way to minimize aerosols and pathogens from reaching those areas, including the exposure button used in dental imaging. Surface barriers are not required

Answer Key and Explanations

for use in dentistry; each office determines its use/nonuse of surface barriers and what types of surface barriers to use or if they prefer to use disinfectants in the operatories after patient care instead. When surface barriers are used and remain intact during a dental procedure, the dental staff is not required to disinfect the area under the barriers because it was not exposed to aerosols due to the protection that the surface barrier provides.

63. D: The federal Consumer-Patient Radiation Health and Safety Act requires that all persons who operate x-ray machinery to produce dental radiographs are properly trained and certified. The *Journal of the American Dental Association* (JADA) is filled with useful information regarding the practice of dentistry in the United States. The Occupational Safety and Health Administration (OSHA) is a federal agency that regulates workplace safety and health. The Food and Drug Administration (FDA) is a regulating agency in the United States that promotes proper health and human services through laws and state regulations.

64. C: Cotton rolls can aid in the placement of an image receptor when the patient has edentulous areas in their oral cavity. If teeth are missing on one arch during a bitewing image, the cotton rolls can serve as a device to help hold the bitewing tab into place, allowing for maximum stability of the image receptor. The dental auxiliary does not need to use cotton roll holders when placing cotton rolls in a patient's oral cavity because the metal from the holder may distort the image.

65. D: There are several methods that can be used to sterilize patient care items used in dental imaging with the steam autoclave being the method that, when used correctly, can provide sterilization of items using water steam under pressure. This method can also prevent corrosion of patient care items, and when the cycle is run to completion, it will produce items that are dry in their packaging and are ready for storage. Unsaturated chemical vapor sterilization methods use a chemical vapor to sterilize instruments under pressure. Instruments must be dry prior to using this method; otherwise, corrosion may occur. Both forced air and rapid transfer are types of dry heat sterilization that use dry environments to sterilize items and produce items that are dry after each cycle.

66. D: A developing fetus would be the most sensitive to the effects of radiation because a fetus is an accumulation of cells that are constantly undergoing cellular division and replication. If these cells are damaged at this stage, they may produce other damaged cells that will affect the developing fetus. More radiation damage occurs in cells that are sensitive to radiation and are rapidly dividing, such as those of a developing fetus.

67. B: The XCP device, used in dentistry as a beam alignment device and a receptor holder, is an example of an engineering control because it is a physical piece of equipment used to provide operator safety. This device can save the dental provider from unnecessary radiation as well as prevent risks of exposure that can occur when the dental provider must manipulate an imaging sensor inside a patient's mouth during dental imaging. The practice of using an XCP device in dental imaging is an example of a work practice control that may be required in some dental practices but optional in others.

68. C: The collimator is a part of the tubehead. It is a metal disc made out of lead located near the position-indicating device (PID). The x-ray beam passes through the collimator. It allows the beam to exit through a 2-inch opening. It forms the size and the shape of the x-ray beam. A rectangular shape helps to limit the amount of radiation exposure the patient receives. There is a filter located within the PID that filters out the unusable wavelengths, such as the longer waves that are not used for dental radiographs.

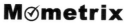

69. B: The American Academy of Oral and Maxillofacial Radiology recommends using the paralleling technique, which provides the dentist with the most accurate image with the least amount of distortion. This recommendation stems from the theory that if the dental film is placed parallel to the long axis of the tooth during exposure, this will provide the least possible means of distortion of the tooth being radiographed.

70. D: As a dental assistant, it is important to be able to interpret radiographs and identify structures appropriately. Structures that are visualized as radiopaque are dense structures that block the x-rays from passing through them. There may be a range of radiopacity; they may be seen as white to light gray on the film. Structures that will be viewed as radiopaque include enamel, dentin, cementum, lamina dura, interradicular bone, and interdental bone. Other radiopaque areas will include the hard palate, nasal septum, and maxillary tuberosity. Radiolucent areas on dental radiographs will appear within the range of dark gray to black. The structures are not as dense as the radiopaque structures and the x-rays are able to penetrate the structures to some degree. Structures that will be viewed as radiolucent include the pulp chamber, pulp canals, periodontal ligament, mandibular canal, lingual foramen, and mandibular foramen.

71. B: A pathogen is a type of microorganism that is capable of causing disease. Bacteria and protozoa can be pathogenic in nature, but not always. For instance, there are healthy types of bacteria found in our food or in the normal flora of our gastrointestinal tract. There are not healthy types of pathogens that exist—all pathogens can cause disease. A biofilm is a type of layer composed of bacterial colonies that form together. A biofilm may be found within dental unit water lines and is composed of a variety of different microbes including pathogens but is not pathogenic itself.

72. C: Legally, dental images, as part of the patient's dental record, are the property of the dentist. The patient, patient's authorized caretaker, and the insurance company are able to review, or have a copy of, the dental images, once authorized for release by the patient. Although the patient or the insurance company has paid for the services to have the images taken, the images legally belong to the provider.

73. B: All of the structures listed would appear radiolucent (in varying degrees) on a processed dental periapical x-ray EXCEPT the nasal septum. This anatomical landmark would appear more radiopaque than radiolucent. The nasal septum is composed of dense bone that prohibits the x-ray beam from successfully going through the film completely due to the thickness of the bone. An image would be created by the exposure in this area, but the resulting radiograph will indicate a radiopacity in the area of this anatomical landmark rather than a radiolucency.

74. B: When possible, an XCP device should be precleaned using the ultrasonic machine, which uses high-frequency sound waves to efficiently and effectively vibrate bioburden off of instruments. This, along with the use of ultrasonic products that have enzymatic or antimicrobial activity, is the best option for precleaning instruments in dentistry. The holding solution is used to prevent bioburden from drying onto instruments and is not a method of precleaning. Hand scrubbing is the least desirable cleaning method due to the risk of occupational injury when scrubbing sharp instruments. The instrument washing machine works similarly to a household dishwasher and serves as a thermal disinfector for instruments; it does not use high-frequency sound waves to loosen and remove debris.

75. A: It is not acceptable for the dental auxiliary to hold an image receptor in a patient's mouth under any circumstances. This is because this action may result in unnecessary exposure to both

Answer Key and Explanations

113

primary and secondary or scatter radiation to the dental auxiliary, which does not follow the ALARA principle.

76. C: Intermediate-level disinfectants are used when disinfecting clinical contact surfaces, including the dental tubehead and dental operatory after dental imaging. This level of disinfectant has the ability to destroy a wide range of microbes while having the ability to prevent extensive damage to dental equipment, making it very common in dentistry. A high-level disinfectant is not required for use when disinfecting clinical contact surfaces, and a sterilant is recommended for use only for reusable heat-sensitive items and by immersion only. Low-level disinfectants are recommended for cleaning and disinfecting floors, walls, and other noncritical surfaces.

77. A: When mounting processed radiographs, the anatomical landmark that can assist you in mounting the mandibular premolar periapical is the mental foramen. The genial tubercles and the lingual foramen are anatomical landmarks located in the lingual mandibular anterior area. The premolar is considered a posterior tooth and would not be associated with any of the mandibular anterior landmarks for proper identification or mounting. The maxillary sinus is an anatomical landmark that is associated with mounting the maxillary anterior and posterior periapicals.

78. D: Disproportionate changes in the size of an image on a processed radiograph are caused by excessive or insufficient vertical angulation. The inability to see between the contacts of the teeth is the result of improper horizontal angulation. The size of the film will only directly relate to disproportionate changes in the processed radiograph if too small of a film was used to perhaps see the apex of a tooth.

79. B: The function of the kilovoltage (kVp) peak selector is to control the degree of penetration from the x-ray beam. The normal kVp of a dental radiograph machine is 60-90 kVp. The 90 kVp setting is used for an image with a lower degree of contrast. This image will contain more gray shades and has a lower exposure time. A 60 kVp is used for an image with a higher degree of contrast. It has fewer gray shades in the image and more definitive light and dark areas. The exposure time is slightly longer. Dentists will have their own individual preferences for the kilovoltage peak selector that is used for most images.

80. D: When considering what image to take in order to obtain the best view of facial growth, facial trauma and disease, or developmental abnormalities that may occur in the oral cavity or cranium, the lateral cephalometric projection is the top choice. This is due to the large 8 x 10 cassette that is used to capture this image and also how the vertical and horizontal angulations are set up when exposing this image. This image is commonly taken in orthodontic offices and used to allow the dentist to trace the anticipated growth of the mandible and maxilla as braces are considered for a patient.

How to Overcome Test Anxiety

Just the thought of taking a test is enough to make most people a little nervous. A test is an important event that can have a long-term impact on your future, so it's important to take it seriously and it's natural to feel anxious about performing well. But just because anxiety is normal, that doesn't mean that it's helpful in test taking, or that you should simply accept it as part of your life. Anxiety can have a variety of effects. These effects can be mild, like making you feel slightly nervous, or severe, like blocking your ability to focus or remember even a simple detail.

If you experience test anxiety—whether severe or mild—it's important to know how to beat it. To discover this, first you need to understand what causes test anxiety.

Causes of Test Anxiety

While we often think of anxiety as an uncontrollable emotional state, it can actually be caused by simple, practical things. One of the most common causes of test anxiety is that a person does not feel adequately prepared for their test. This feeling can be the result of many different issues such as poor study habits or lack of organization, but the most common culprit is time management. Starting to study too late, failing to organize your study time to cover all of the material, or being distracted while you study will mean that you're not well prepared for the test. This may lead to cramming the night before, which will cause you to be physically and mentally exhausted for the test. Poor time management also contributes to feelings of stress, fear, and hopelessness as you realize you are not well prepared but don't know what to do about it.

Other times, test anxiety is not related to your preparation for the test but comes from unresolved fear. This may be a past failure on a test, or poor performance on tests in general. It may come from comparing yourself to others who seem to be performing better or from the stress of living up to expectations. Anxiety may be driven by fears of the future—how failure on this test would affect your educational and career goals. These fears are often completely irrational, but they can still negatively impact your test performance.

Elements of Test Anxiety

As mentioned earlier, test anxiety is considered to be an emotional state, but it has physical and mental components as well. Sometimes you may not even realize that you are suffering from test anxiety until you notice the physical symptoms. These can include trembling hands, rapid heartbeat, sweating, nausea, and tense muscles. Extreme anxiety may lead to fainting or vomiting. Obviously, any of these symptoms can have a negative impact on testing. It is important to recognize them as soon as they begin to occur so that you can address the problem before it damages your performance.

The mental components of test anxiety include trouble focusing and inability to remember learned information. During a test, your mind is on high alert, which can help you recall information and stay focused for an extended period of time. However, anxiety interferes with your mind's natural processes, causing you to blank out, even on the questions you know well. The strain of testing during anxiety makes it difficult to stay focused, especially on a test that may take several hours. Extreme anxiety can take a huge mental toll, making it difficult not only to recall test information but even to understand the test questions or pull your thoughts together.

Effects of Test Anxiety

Test anxiety is like a disease—if left untreated, it will get progressively worse. Anxiety leads to poor performance, and this reinforces the feelings of fear and failure, which in turn lead to poor performances on subsequent tests. It can grow from a mild nervousness to a crippling condition. If allowed to progress, test anxiety can have a big impact on your schooling, and consequently on your future.

Test anxiety can spread to other parts of your life. Anxiety on tests can become anxiety in any stressful situation, and blanking on a test can turn into panicking in a job situation. But fortunately, you don't have to let anxiety rule your testing and determine your grades. There are a number of relatively simple steps you can take to move past anxiety and function normally on a test and in the rest of life.

Physical Steps for Beating Test Anxiety

While test anxiety is a serious problem, the good news is that it can be overcome. It doesn't have to control your ability to think and remember information. While it may take time, you can begin taking steps today to beat anxiety.

Just as your first hint that you may be struggling with anxiety comes from the physical symptoms, the first step to treating it is also physical. Rest is crucial for having a clear, strong mind. If you are tired, it is much easier to give in to anxiety. But if you establish good sleep habits, your body and mind will be ready to perform optimally, without the strain of exhaustion. Additionally, sleeping well helps you to retain information better, so you're more likely to recall the answers when you see the test questions.

Getting good sleep means more than going to bed on time. It's important to allow your brain time to relax. Take study breaks from time to time so it doesn't get overworked, and don't study right before bed. Take time to rest your mind before trying to rest your body, or you may find it difficult to fall asleep.

Along with sleep, other aspects of physical health are important in preparing for a test. Good nutrition is vital for good brain function. Sugary foods and drinks may give a burst of energy but this burst is followed by a crash, both physically and emotionally. Instead, fuel your body with protein and vitamin-rich foods.

Also, drink plenty of water. Dehydration can lead to headaches and exhaustion, especially if your brain is already under stress from the rigors of the test. Particularly if your test is a long one, drink water during the breaks. And if possible, take an energy-boosting snack to eat between sections.

Along with sleep and diet, a third important part of physical health is exercise. Maintaining a steady workout schedule is helpful, but even taking 5-minute study breaks to walk can help get your blood pumping faster and clear your head. Exercise also releases endorphins, which contribute to a positive feeling and can help combat test anxiety.

When you nurture your physical health, you are also contributing to your mental health. If your body is healthy, your mind is much more likely to be healthy as well. So take time to rest, nourish your body with healthy food and water, and get moving as much as possible. Taking these physical steps will make you stronger and more able to take the mental steps necessary to overcome test anxiety.

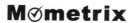

Mental Steps for Beating Test Anxiety

Working on the mental side of test anxiety can be more challenging, but as with the physical side, there are clear steps you can take to overcome it. As mentioned earlier, test anxiety often stems from lack of preparation, so the obvious solution is to prepare for the test. Effective studying may be the most important weapon you have for beating test anxiety, but you can and should employ several other mental tools to combat fear.

First, boost your confidence by reminding yourself of past success—tests or projects that you aced. If you're putting as much effort into preparing for this test as you did for those, there's no reason you should expect to fail here. Work hard to prepare; then trust your preparation.

Second, surround yourself with encouraging people. It can be helpful to find a study group, but be sure that the people you're around will encourage a positive attitude. If you spend time with others who are anxious or cynical, this will only contribute to your own anxiety. Look for others who are motivated to study hard from a desire to succeed, not from a fear of failure.

Third, reward yourself. A test is physically and mentally tiring, even without anxiety, and it can be helpful to have something to look forward to. Plan an activity following the test, regardless of the outcome, such as going to a movie or getting ice cream.

When you are taking the test, if you find yourself beginning to feel anxious, remind yourself that you know the material. Visualize successfully completing the test. Then take a few deep, relaxing breaths and return to it. Work through the questions carefully but with confidence, knowing that you are capable of succeeding.

Developing a healthy mental approach to test taking will also aid in other areas of life. Test anxiety affects more than just the actual test—it can be damaging to your mental health and even contribute to depression. It's important to beat test anxiety before it becomes a problem for more than testing.

Study Strategy

Being prepared for the test is necessary to combat anxiety, but what does being prepared look like? You may study for hours on end and still not feel prepared. What you need is a strategy for test prep. The next few pages outline our recommended steps to help you plan out and conquer the challenge of preparation.

STEP 1: SCOPE OUT THE TEST

Learn everything you can about the format (multiple choice, essay, etc.) and what will be on the test. Gather any study materials, course outlines, or sample exams that may be available. Not only will this help you to prepare, but knowing what to expect can help to alleviate test anxiety.

STEP 2: MAP OUT THE MATERIAL

Look through the textbook or study guide and make note of how many chapters or sections it has. Then divide these over the time you have. For example, if a book has 15 chapters and you have five days to study, you need to cover three chapters each day. Even better, if you have the time, leave an extra day at the end for overall review after you have gone through the material in depth.

If time is limited, you may need to prioritize the material. Look through it and make note of which sections you think you already have a good grasp on, and which need review. While you are studying, skim quickly through the familiar sections and take more time on the challenging parts.

How to Overcome Test Anxiety

117

Write out your plan so you don't get lost as you go. Having a written plan also helps you feel more in control of the study, so anxiety is less likely to arise from feeling overwhelmed at the amount to cover.

STEP 3: GATHER YOUR TOOLS

Decide what study method works best for you. Do you prefer to highlight in the book as you study and then go back over the highlighted portions? Or do you type out notes of the important information? Or is it helpful to make flashcards that you can carry with you? Assemble the pens, index cards, highlighters, post-it notes, and any other materials you may need so you won't be distracted by getting up to find things while you study.

If you're having a hard time retaining the information or organizing your notes, experiment with different methods. For example, try color-coding by subject with colored pens, highlighters, or post-it notes. If you learn better by hearing, try recording yourself reading your notes so you can listen while in the car, working out, or simply sitting at your desk. Ask a friend to quiz you from your flashcards, or try teaching someone the material to solidify it in your mind.

STEP 4: CREATE YOUR ENVIRONMENT

It's important to avoid distractions while you study. This includes both the obvious distractions like visitors and the subtle distractions like an uncomfortable chair (or a too-comfortable couch that makes you want to fall asleep). Set up the best study environment possible: good lighting and a comfortable work area. If background music helps you focus, you may want to turn it on, but otherwise keep the room quiet. If you are using a computer to take notes, be sure you don't have any other windows open, especially applications like social media, games, or anything else that could distract you. Silence your phone and turn off notifications. Be sure to keep water close by so you stay hydrated while you study (but avoid unhealthy drinks and snacks).

Also, take into account the best time of day to study. Are you freshest first thing in the morning? Try to set aside some time then to work through the material. Is your mind clearer in the afternoon or evening? Schedule your study session then. Another method is to study at the same time of day that you will take the test, so that your brain gets used to working on the material at that time and will be ready to focus at test time.

STEP 5: STUDY!

Once you have done all the study preparation, it's time to settle into the actual studying. Sit down, take a few moments to settle your mind so you can focus, and begin to follow your study plan. Don't give in to distractions or let yourself procrastinate. This is your time to prepare so you'll be ready to fearlessly approach the test. Make the most of the time and stay focused.

Of course, you don't want to burn out. If you study too long you may find that you're not retaining the information very well. Take regular study breaks. For example, taking five minutes out of every hour to walk briskly, breathing deeply and swinging your arms, can help your mind stay fresh.

As you get to the end of each chapter or section, it's a good idea to do a quick review. Remind yourself of what you learned and work on any difficult parts. When you feel that you've mastered the material, move on to the next part. At the end of your study session, briefly skim through your notes again.

But while review is helpful, cramming last minute is NOT. If at all possible, work ahead so that you won't need to fit all your study into the last day. Cramming overloads your brain with more information than it can process and retain, and your tired mind may struggle to recall even

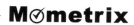
previously learned information when it is overwhelmed with last-minute study. Also, the urgent nature of cramming and the stress placed on your brain contribute to anxiety. You'll be more likely to go to the test feeling unprepared and having trouble thinking clearly.

So don't cram, and don't stay up late before the test, even just to review your notes at a leisurely pace. Your brain needs rest more than it needs to go over the information again. In fact, plan to finish your studies by noon or early afternoon the day before the test. Give your brain the rest of the day to relax or focus on other things, and get a good night's sleep. Then you will be fresh for the test and better able to recall what you've studied.

STEP 6: TAKE A PRACTICE TEST

Many courses offer sample tests, either online or in the study materials. This is an excellent resource to check whether you have mastered the material, as well as to prepare for the test format and environment.

Check the test format ahead of time: the number of questions, the type (multiple choice, free response, etc.), and the time limit. Then create a plan for working through them. For example, if you have 30 minutes to take a 60-question test, your limit is 30 seconds per question. Spend less time on the questions you know well so that you can take more time on the difficult ones.

If you have time to take several practice tests, take the first one open book, with no time limit. Work through the questions at your own pace and make sure you fully understand them. Gradually work up to taking a test under test conditions: sit at a desk with all study materials put away and set a timer. Pace yourself to make sure you finish the test with time to spare and go back to check your answers if you have time.

After each test, check your answers. On the questions you missed, be sure you understand why you missed them. Did you misread the question (tests can use tricky wording)? Did you forget the information? Or was it something you hadn't learned? Go back and study any shaky areas that the practice tests reveal.

Taking these tests not only helps with your grade, but also aids in combating test anxiety. If you're already used to the test conditions, you're less likely to worry about it, and working through tests until you're scoring well gives you a confidence boost. Go through the practice tests until you feel comfortable, and then you can go into the test knowing that you're ready for it.

Test Tips

On test day, you should be confident, knowing that you've prepared well and are ready to answer the questions. But aside from preparation, there are several test day strategies you can employ to maximize your performance.

First, as stated before, get a good night's sleep the night before the test (and for several nights before that, if possible). Go into the test with a fresh, alert mind rather than staying up late to study.

Try not to change too much about your normal routine on the day of the test. It's important to eat a nutritious breakfast, but if you normally don't eat breakfast at all, consider eating just a protein bar. If you're a coffee drinker, go ahead and have your normal coffee. Just make sure you time it so that the caffeine doesn't wear off right in the middle of your test. Avoid sugary beverages, and drink enough water to stay hydrated but not so much that you need a restroom break 10 minutes into the test. If your test isn't first thing in the morning, consider going for a walk or doing a light workout before the test to get your blood flowing.

Allow yourself enough time to get ready, and leave for the test with plenty of time to spare so you won't have the anxiety of scrambling to arrive in time. Another reason to be early is to select a good seat. It's helpful to sit away from doors and windows, which can be distracting. Find a good seat, get out your supplies, and settle your mind before the test begins.

When the test begins, start by going over the instructions carefully, even if you already know what to expect. Make sure you avoid any careless mistakes by following the directions.

Then begin working through the questions, pacing yourself as you've practiced. If you're not sure on an answer, don't spend too much time on it, and don't let it shake your confidence. Either skip it and come back later, or eliminate as many wrong answers as possible and guess among the remaining ones. Don't dwell on these questions as you continue—put them out of your mind and focus on what lies ahead.

Be sure to read all of the answer choices, even if you're sure the first one is the right answer. Sometimes you'll find a better one if you keep reading. But don't second-guess yourself if you do immediately know the answer. Your gut instinct is usually right. Don't let test anxiety rob you of the information you know.

If you have time at the end of the test (and if the test format allows), go back and review your answers. Be cautious about changing any, since your first instinct tends to be correct, but make sure you didn't misread any of the questions or accidentally mark the wrong answer choice. Look over any you skipped and make an educated guess.

At the end, leave the test feeling confident. You've done your best, so don't waste time worrying about your performance or wishing you could change anything. Instead, celebrate the successful completion of this test. And finally, use this test to learn how to deal with anxiety even better next time.

> **Review Video: Test Anxiety**
> Visit mometrix.com/academy and enter code: 100340

Important Qualification

Not all anxiety is created equal. If your test anxiety is causing major issues in your life beyond the classroom or testing center, or if you are experiencing troubling physical symptoms related to your anxiety, it may be a sign of a serious physiological or psychological condition. If this sounds like your situation, we strongly encourage you to seek professional help.

Additional Bonus Material

Due to our efforts to try to keep this book to a manageable length, we've created a link that will give you access to all of your additional bonus material:

mometrix.com/bonus948/danbrhs